Flavien NDE AZER

ANESTHESIA IN SHOCKED PATIENTS:

Flavien NDE AZER

ANESTHESIA IN SHOCKED PATIENTS:

A contextual study of obstetrical and digestive emergencies

ScienciaScripts

Imprint

Cover image: www.ingimage.com

This book is a translation from the original published under ISBN 978-620-6-72134-5.

Publisher:
Sciencia Scripts
is a trademark of
Dodo Books Indian Ocean Ltd. and OmniScriptum S.R.L publishing group

120 High Road, East Finchley, London, N2 9ED, United Kingdom
Str. Armeneasca 28/1, office 1, Chisinau MD-2012, Republic of Moldova, Europe
Printed at: see last page
ISBN: 978-620-8-19474-1

DEDICACES

A

- ❖ my dear wife, **Jacqueline NDE**: thank you for your constant concern for me.

ACKNOWLEDGEMENTS

❖ To Professor **Jacqueline ZE MINKANDE** and Professor **Fidèle BINAM**, for their teaching and constant encouragement to complete this difficult but fascinating training for the Master's degree in Health Sciences, option Anesthesia-Resuscitation.

❖ To Doctor **Etienne PENLAP** and **Madame** for organizing, co-directing and monitoring this work.

❖ To Doctor **Benjamin Alexandre NKOUM**, Director of the Centre Supérieur des Sciences de la Santé, you are the fountain of knowledge.

❖ To Dr **DJIMEFO** for the bio-statistical support of this very laborious work.

❖ To Dr. **NGAYAP** for his profound understanding of the students' problem.

❖ We would like to express our deepest sympathy to Mr **Mathurin IPACK IPACK**, coordinator of the Master's program in Anaesthesia and Intensive Care.

❖ To my colleagues in the first class of the Master in Anaesthesia-Resuscitation for the collaboration and mutual support that have characterized us over the past two years.

We would like to express our gratitude to :

❖ Docteur **Pierre MALONGTE**, Docteur **DJIMEFO**, Docteur **BASSEGUE**, Madame **Julienne EKODI**, Monsieur **NOUMSSI**, Monsieur **Etienne KIMESSOUKIE**, Monsieur **Henri BITHA**, Monsieur **MBA Maurice**, in short all the teachers at UCAC (Université Catholique d'Afrique Centrale).

Our gratitude goes to

❖ Mifi District Head of Health, Dr **Daniel MABAPGOUAP** and his colleagues, members of MUPERSADIM (Mutuelle des Personnels de Santé du District de la Mifi) and ARFOSAPDISMI (Association des Responsables des Formations Sanitaires Privées du District de la Mifi).

❖ All the supervisors at the training sites: Service Majors, Unit Managers and Residents.

❖ To Mrs **Marceline NZIE** for her advice, patience and availability.

❖ To all my brothers and sisters, relatives, friends and acquaintances, we thank you for your generosity and solicitude in supporting this work. May God bless you all!

ABBREVIATIONS

ASA	=	American of Society Anesthesiologists
ASP	=	Abdomen Sans Préparation
BPCO	=	Bronchopneunopathie Chronique et Obstructive
CG	=	Culot Globulaire
ECG	=	Electrocardiogramme
GEUR	=	Grossesse Extra-utérine Rompue
HA	=	Hypovolémie Absolue
HBPM	=	Héparine de Bas Poids Moléculaire
HGOPY	=	Hôpital Gynéco Obstétrique et Pédiatrique de Yaoundé
HR	=	Hypovolémie Relative
IADE	=	Infirmier Anesthésiste Diplômé d'Etat
IDE	=	Infirmier Diplômé d'Etat
MAR	=	Médecin Anesthésiste Réanimateur
NFS	=	Numération Formule Sanguine
OAP	=	Œdème Aigu du Poumon
P.O	=	Pouvoir Oncotique
PA	=	Pression Artérielle
PAS	=	Pression Artérielle Systolique
PEEP	=	Pression Positive en Fin d'Expiration
PFC	=	Plasma Frais Congelé
PSE	=	Pousse Seringue Electrique
PVC	=	Pression Veineuse Centrale
RAI	=	Recherche d'Agglutinines Irrégulières
RAS	=	Résistances Artérielles Systémiques
SDRA	=	Syndrome de Détresse Respiratoire Aigue de l'Adulte
SG	=	Soluté Glucosé
SP	=	Sérum Physiologique
SPO_2	=	Saturation Artérielle en Oxygène
ST	=	Sus-décalage du Segment
TCK	=	Temps de Céphaline Kaolin
TP	=	Temps de Prothrombine
VD	=	Ventricule Droit
VG	=	Ventricule Gauche

SUMMARY

Hypovolemic shock is a frequent cause of mortality and morbidity in emergency departments, intensive care units and operating theatres. This is particularly true in poor countries, where it must be borne in mind that a large proportion of the population arrive at hospital late [2], not to mention inadequate technical facilities and limited monitoring resources.

The aim of this work was to describe the epidemiological profile, means and methods of anesthetic management of shocked patients in the context of obstetric and digestive emergencies. We carried out a retrospective and descriptive study on the records of patients operated on for obstetric and digestive emergencies, during the period from January 1er 2011 to January 31 2012 at the Yaoundé Gyneco-obstetric and Pediatric Hospital. Our work lasted four months. The number of patients selected for the study was 144.

The parameters studied were: (age, anesthetic risk, anesthetic technique, preoperative hemodynamic status, degree of urgency, venous line quality (type of venous line used, number of venous lines placed; caliber of catheters used), parameters monitored intraoperatively (ECG, PANI, SPao2, diuresis, temperature...intraoperative blood loss, intraoperative monitoring, anesthetic drugs used for anesthetic induction, anesthetic drugs used for anesthetic maintenance, intraoperative hemodynamic variations through intraoperative variations in systolic blood pressure (SBP) and heart rate (HR), quality of filling solutions and blood products used, duration of anesthesia (time between anesthetic induction and discharge from the operating room), duration of the procedure (time between incision and parietal closure), intraoperative incidents and accidents, prescription of postoperative instructions (effective drafting of the postoperative prescription, postoperative check-ups prescribed, prescription of LMWH for prophylaxis), patient outcome (morbidity ; mortality)).

The essential pathologies that caught our attention were listed and categorized. For obstetric emergencies, they included ruptured ectopic pregnancies, hemorrhagic placenta previa and retroplacental hematomas, hemostasis hysterectomy, uterine rupture and hemoperitoneum. Digestive emergencies included intestinal occlusions and peritonitis.

GEUR was the main pathology likely to induce hemodynamic instability.

Half the patients were aged between 25 and 35.

The majority of patients were ASA I or II, and 88.89% of procedures were extreme emergencies.

The parameters monitored were: ECG, non-invasive blood pressure, heart rate, oxygen saturation and diuresis.

GA was the main anesthetic technique and 65.28% of patients were hemodynamically unstable.

No deaths in the operating room.

Management influenced by the absence of certain anaesthetic and blood products.

In view of the results of our survey and with a view to making our contribution to the management of shocked patients in the context of obstetric and digestive emergencies, we draw up the following proposals:

Ministry of Public Health:

- organize regular in-service training for staff
- provide each referral hospital with an emergency kit for the immediate care of shocked patients in obstetric and digestive emergencies
- Supply hospitals with etomidate and blood banks with platelet concentrates and fresh frozen plasma.

To HGOPY General Management:

- organize anesthetic record keeping
- set up a computerized archiving system to provide a good database for future studies
- Maintain the monitoring equipment system

We are also encouraging a similar prospective study.

KEYWORDS
Hemodynamics - Epidemiology - Profile - Emergencies - Shock

CONTENTS

INTRODUCTION

Hypovolemic shock is one of the most common problems faced by anesthetists, whether before anesthesia, during surgery or afterwards.

Absolute hypovolemia can be defined as a reduction in blood mass [3]. It may result from haemorrhage, reduced plasma mass due to hydrosodium deficiency, or extravasation of water and sodium to interstitial tissues.

The term relative hypovolemia refers to situations where an increase in the vascular bed leads to a decrease in venous blood return to the heart. Relative hypovolemia is involved in the pathophysiology of septic shock and anaphylactic shock during general or locoregional anesthesia [3].

The aim of vascular filling is to correct absolute or relative volume deficits.

Hypovolemia is a frequent cause of mortality and morbidity in emergency departments, intensive care units and operating theatres. This is particularly true in poor countries, where it must be borne in mind that a large proportion of the population arrives at hospital late [26], not to mention the inadequate technical facilities and limited monitoring resources.

With the aim of making our contribution to the anesthetic management of hypovolemic patients, we proposed to work on shocked patients operated on in the context of obstetric emergencies due to hemorrhage (GEUR, hemorrhagic placenta previa, retroplacental hematoma, hemostasis hysterectomy, uterine rupture, postoperative hemoperitoneum) or 3eme sector formation (intestinal occlusions and peritonitis).

CHAPTER 1: ISSUES

1-1- PROBLEM STATEMENT

Hypovolemia, whether absolute or relative, is an emergency situation. It occurs in a variety of surgical pathologies, the pathophysiological mechanisms of which are either bleeding, dehydration or the formation of a third sector.

Hypovolemia leads to reduced tissue perfusion. If not promptly managed, it leads to cell death and irreversible multivisceral failure if effective treatment is not instituted. In sub-Saharan Africa, patients consult their doctor late. Delayed diagnosis and lack of adequate management resources are compounded by significant morbidity and mortality [39].

In an emergency, it is important to rapidly identify situations that may lead to hypovolemia, and to make a rapid diagnosis so as to institute monitoring and prompt, appropriate management.

In our underdeveloped countries, the management of sub-hospital emergencies is still in its infancy, and the technical resources available in hospitals are highly inadequate. It is in this difficult context that we propose to carry out this study on anesthesia in shocked patients in the context of obstetric and digestive emergencies, in order to contribute to the management of emergencies in underprivileged areas.

1-2- RESEARCH HYPOTHESIS

Anesthetic management of shocked patients in obstetric and digestive emergencies in hospitals in poor countries is difficult for a number of reasons that need to be identified.

1-3- RESEARCH QUESTION

What are the epidemiological profiles of shocked patients in the context of obstetric and digestive emergencies managed at the Yaoundé Gyneco-Obstetric and Pediatric Hospital?

CHAPTER 2: OBJECTIVES

2-1- GENERAL OBJECTIVE

Describe the epidemiological profile of patients, and the means and methods of anesthetic management of shocked patients in obstetric and digestive emergencies.

2-2- SPECIFIC OBJECTIVES

- Identify surgical pathologies leading to shock in obstetrical and digestive emergencies
- Determine the epidemiological profile of patients
- Determine patients' anesthetic risk and degree of urgency
- Record incidents and accidents (collapses, hypotension, etc.)
- Describe anesthetic technique and intraoperative hemodynamic variations
- Determining patient outcomes

CHAPTER 3: LITERATURE REVIEW

3-1- HYPOVOLEMIA

3-1-1- General and Definition

Hypovolemic shock results from a decrease in circulating blood mass, the main consequence of which is a drop in venous return and cardiac output. There are several types of hypovolemia, which may be associated [26].

True hypovolemia: This may be due to hemorrhage, plasma leakage (extensive burns, edema) or abundant fluid losses from the digestive or urinary tract, or the creation of a third sector [3,67].

Relative hypovolemia. This is the consequence of an increase in the capacity of the vascular system, the very type of which is anaphylactic shock.

3-1-2- Pathophysiology of hypovolemic shock

The reduction in circulating blood mass leads to a drop in venous return. This decrease in venous return is responsible for a drop in cardiac output, and arterial hypotension. The extent of arterial hypotension depends both on the extent of blood volume reduction and on the effectiveness of compensatory mechanisms, which are diminished by anemia, previous hypovolemia, heart failure or anesthesia. Beta blocker or vasodilator treatment also "alters" compensatory mechanisms [51].

3-1-3- Compensating mechanisms

They rely initially on the response of the sympathetic nervous system. A drop in blood pressure stimulates the baroreflex. The intense sympathetic reaction, with the release of adrenalin and noradrenalin, leads to a significant increase in systemic arterial resistance (SAR). Vasoconstriction is the main response to hypovolemia. There is thus an increase in S.A.R., although this increase is not uniform throughout the body, with certain so-called privileged territories (heart, coronary arteries, central nervous system, kidney, etc.) being preserved to the detriment of muscles, skin and mesentery. Renal circulation is vasoconstricted only when blood spoliation exceeds 30% of circulating blood volume, resulting in oliguria.

Secondary mechanisms for reconstituting plasma volume include fluid transfer from the interstitial to the capillary vascular sector, increased supply of lymphatic albumin to the vascular sector via the thoracic duct, and reabsorption of water and salt by aldosterone secretion.

In the late phase, tissue perfusion is impaired, leading to hypoxia with anaerobic metabolism and metabolic lactic acidosis. Tissue damage also affects the viscera: renal failure with oliguria, lesion-type PAO, digestive ischemia, liver failure, myocardial depression. Ischemic cells release a large number of vasoactive substances that reduce venous return and increase capillary permeability [51].

3-1-4 Diagnosis

3-1-4-1 Positive diagnosis

. Clinical examination

- Anamnesis

- Past history

These are: medical - surgical - gynecological - family - allergological - toxicological - transiusional - anesthesiological - therapeutic.

- Physical examination

It includes inspection, palpation, percussion and auscultation.

The picture combines hypotension **with** signs of altered organ perfusion.

The diagnosis is made when :

- systolic blood pressure below 90 with pinched differential or collapsed or impenetrable.

- sinus tachycardia (over 90 beats per minute) with a rapid, thready pulse that's hard to catch,

- neuropsychological disorders ranging from simple drowsiness to confusion with agitation, anxiety and even coma.

- vasoconstriction of the skin, characterized by paleness of the integuments and mucous membranes, mottling initially limited to the knees and then extending to the thighs and abdomen, coldness and cyanosis of the extremities, and a capillary recoloration time greater than 2 seconds.

- tachypnea greater than 20 cycles per minute.

- intense thirst and constant oligoanuria of less than 20ml/h or 0.5ml/kg/h.

The major danger is to underestimate hypovolemia and neglect its management.

- Biological tests

- A complete blood count (CBC) to look for hyper leukocytosis, anemia and thrombocytopenia.

- Blood group and rhesus for preparation of a possible blood transfusion,

- Investigation of coagulation disorders through platelet count, prothrombin rate (PT) and partial thromboplastin rate (PTR).

- Renal assessment: urea, creatinine, ionogram

- Blood gases and arterial lactates in search of tissue hypoxia resulting in the development of anaerobic metabolism.

- Morphological and electro-physiological examinations

- Electrocardiogram: observation of the tracing enables monitoring of variations in heart rate, rhythm and conduction disorders, and cardiac distress with ST segment modification (sub-shift).

- No-preparation abdomen (NPA) or abdomino-pelvic ultrasound for abdominal or pelvic abnormalities

3-1-4-2 Aetiological diagnosis

- Non-hemorrhagic hypovolemia

- Dehydration

They are linked to hydro-sodium losses of digestive, renal or cutaneous origin [46]. Digestive disorders are the most frequent, with vomiting and diarrhea. Renal losses come next, with some nephropathy and osmotic polyuria. Skin loss from extensive burns, accompanied by major protein loss, is the third most common cause. We exclude relative hypovolemia secondary to intense vasodilation, sometimes associated with plasma leakage as in anaphylactic and septic shock [46].

- The third sector

For the anaesthetist, however, the problem most often encountered is that of the "3^{e} sector", to use Randall's term (F.D. Moore's sequestred oedema). This is the accumulation of fluids in an area temporarily excluded from exchanges. This intense fluid loss is at the expense of extra-cellular fluids, and the quantity thus subtracted can be major, critically reducing blood volume and interstitial fluid (51]. The best-known circumstances are intestinal obstruction and burns.

- Hemorrhagic hypovolemia

Hemorrhage, most often traumatic, can be external (vascular wound, scalp wound, epistaxis) or internal (hemothorax, hemoperitoneum, retroperitoneal hematoma). Outside a traumatic context, it is most often internal (digestive or gynaecological bleeding) or vascular [47].

3-1-5 Management of hypovolemia

3-1-5-1 Purpose

- Stopping bleeding
- Correction and prevention of complications

3-1-5-2 Resources

Non-medicinal means: suture of a vessel, splenectomy for hemostasis, trimming of a liver wound, cure of an ectopic pregnancy, maintenance of blood volume [35, 46].

- Anti-shock pants

It compresses subdiaphragmatic arterial vessels, leading to an increase in RAS, has a haemostatic effect on injured vessels, and mobilizes venous blood from the capacitive system [26].

- Preserving venous return
- A malleable stretcher or resuscitation bed can be used to perform a Trendelenburg, where elevation of the lower limbs temporarily mobilizes 500 to 1000ml of blood to the superior vena cava territory. It is in this latter position that cardiac output is increased the most.
- Oxygen therapy: helps maintain hemodynamic balance.

- Medicinal means

- Catecholamines

They have little use in the initial phase of pure hypovolemic shock. In fact, during hypovolemic shock, the vascular system adapts to hypovolemia through intense vasoconstriction mediated by the sympathetic nervous system and adrenaline secretion by the adrenal medulla. There is a complex vascular redistribution that preserves certain territories, such as the brain, coronary arteries, kidney and liver. Prescribing amines may increase vasoconstriction in territories that were previously preserved. Acute hypovolemia is characterized by a mismatch between content and container. Myocardial contractility is normal or moderately increased.

Nevertheless, catecholamines have major indications: in the event of cardiac arrest due to defibrillation, in association with major volemic expansion.

At anesthetic induction when there is a severe drop in blood pressure. whenever perfusion of noble organs is threatened.

The drug chosen first is dopamine.

In the late phase, two phenomena occur which may justify the use of catecholamines: a decrease in the effect of sympathetic stimulation, and myocardial depression [2].

- Catecholamines are used in conjunction with vascular filling; ephedrine, for example, boosts myocardial contractility and induces vasoconstriction, leading to an increase in blood pressure.

- Filling solutions

* Various filling solutions.

There are two main types: crystalloids and colloids. PFC and CG blood products, as well as albumin, should not be considered as volume expanders [48, 49].

Isotonic crystalloid solutions: 0.9% NaCI, Ringer lactate. They are characterized by low volemic expansion: 200 to 300ml per liter of infused solution. Early mobilization of interstitial albumin, absence of anaphylactic effects **and** low cost make them attractive. However, in the event of severe blood pressure collapse or even shock, macromolecules are preferred.

* Colloids

Dextrans:

They are no longer used in emergencies due to their anaphylactoid risk [59]. Indeed, Promit* must be administered a few minutes before the infusion of a plasmacair dextran. High-molecular-weight dextrans, such as dextrans 40, have disappeared, as they were in any case contraindicated in hypovolemic renal failure.

Fluid gelatins:

Their immediate volemic expansion capacity is slightly less than the volume infused, and their plasma half-life is around 4 hours. They all carry a risk of anaphylactoid reaction. They are made from bovine gelatin. Given the problems posed by prions, it is currently more prudent not to use them.

Hydroxv-ethyl starches:

They achieve a volemic expansion slightly greater than the volume infused (1.5 times), with a duration of action of 12 to 24 hours. They have no deleterious effect on the kidney, and practically no anaphylactoid reaction, but daily volumes are limited, as they may cause blood crase disorders.

Blood derivatives

- PFCs :

They pose the problem of viral and immunological pathologies. Their use is reserved for the correction of blood crase disorders induced by severe acute haemorrhage. They play an important role in the treatment of DIC.

Albumin: reserved for cases of massive albumin loss, burns, postoperative peritoneal carcinosis, treatment of ascites in association with diuretics [35].

In the event of massive transfusions, coagulation disorders may occur, due to a reduction in fibrinogen and platelets. In order to avoid these disorders, the transfusion strategy is now perfectly codified by the so-called Lundsgaard-Hansen scheme (see diagram below). For blood losses of up to 20% of total mass, colloids and crystalloids are sufficient. For a loss of between 20% and 50% of the total blood mass, red blood cells and colloids should be given. For losses between 50 and 100%, albumin is added. Above 100%, platelet concentrates, coagulation factors and albumin are added. Naturally, the prescriber will adapt this regimen to each individual case.

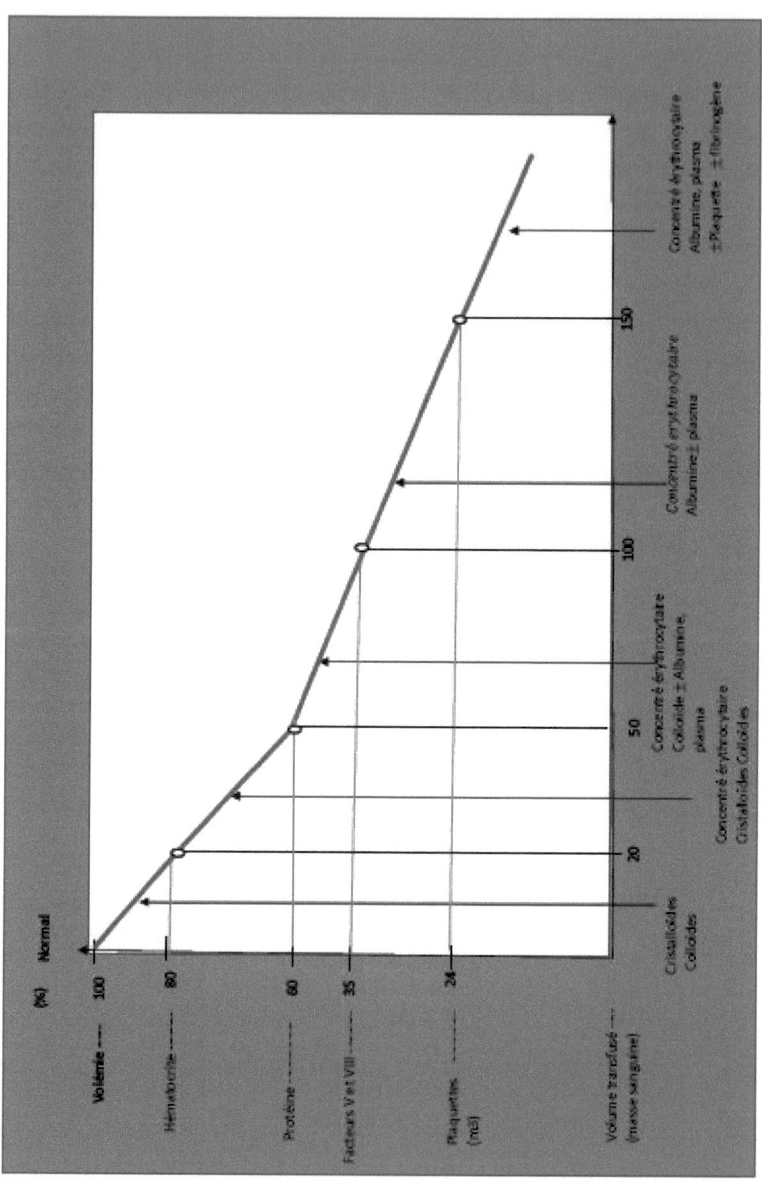

Figure 1 Hemorrhage compensation according to LUNSDGAARD HANSEN (DALENS; 2001).

- Hypertonic crystalloids :

They are rarely used in France. The most common are 5% and 7.5% NaCI, at low cost. They have an expander effect: they have the advantage of reducing intracranial pressure and intrapulmonary water [35].

- Monitoring resources

- The multiparameter monitor
- Precordial stethoscope
- a second-hand watch
- tensiometer
- arterial catheter and invasive blood pressure monitoring equipment
- urinary catheter and graduated urine collector
- nasogastric tube with graduated manifold
- Vacuum cleaner with graduated jar in working order
- Saturometer
- Thermometer
- Tape measure to measure abdominal circumference if necessary

3-1-5-3 Processing method

- General measurement

It consists of installing the patient and getting him/her into condition:

- Safe 16- and 18-gauge venous lines for good volume expansion.
- Good-calibre nasogastric tube
- Nasal oxygen (3 to 6 liters per minute) for good ventilation
- Urinary catheter to monitor urine output and diuresis.
- Specific measures Vascular filling.

Reliable 14- and 16-gauge approaches are required at the bend of the elbow, in the external jugular vein, or with a femoral stent. It is sometimes useful to have one line in the superior vena cava and another in the inferior vena cava, especially in polytrauma patients. As far as possible, rewarming should not be forgotten.

For gastric protection, we administer antacids, anti-H_2 , proton pump inhibitors.

- Prevent thrombo-embolic diseases by using low-molecular-weight heparins such as lovenox* 2000 to 4000 IU subcutaneously per day in a single injection, and wearing compression stockings.

- Hydration

It is carried out through crystalloids (Ringer lactate, saline solution) depending on the degree of dehydration.

Transfusion: according to the French Health Products Safety Agency 2002, the table summarizing the symptoms observed according to the extent of blood loss and not the results of clinical studies is as follows:

Table I Symptomatology according to the extent of blood loss in adults.

Blood loss (ml)	750	800-1500	1500-2000	Over 2000
Diastolic blood pressure (mm Hg)	Unchanged	Normal	Decreased	Very low
Systolic blood pressure (mm Hg)	Unchanged	Augmented	Decreased	Very low or unobstructed
Pulse (minute)	Moderate tachycardia	100-120	Above 120 (low)	Above 120 (very low)
Hair coloring	Normal	Slow (over 2 sec)	Slow (over 2 sec)	Undetectable
Respiratory frequency	Normal	Normal	Tachypnea (above 20/min)	Tachypnea (sup *i* 20/min)
Urine flow (ml/h)	Sup à 30	20-30	10-20	0-10
Ends	Normal	Pale	Pale	Pale and cold
Color	Normal	Pale	Pale	Grey
Awareness	Normal	Anxiety or aggressiveness	Anxiety or aggressiveness or impaired	Altered or comatose

Symptoms associated with volume and/or red blood cell depletion include syncope, dyspnea, tachycardia, angina, postural hypotension and transient ischemic attack [37].

While waiting for blood to arrive, colloids (geloplasma, gelatin) are administered.

Oxygen transport cannot be maintained when hematocrit is below 20%; below 20%, metabolic lactic acidosis occurs, as anaerobic metabolism sets in. It is therefore necessary to group the patient from the outset, take an IAA and start a transfusion depending on the severity of the hemorrhage.

In practice, the minimum threshold for transfusion in the presence of hemorrhage is: hemoglobin 8g/dl or hematocrit 26%, platelet count 50,000 - 75,000 g/dl, fibnogen < 0.8g/l, PT < 30-35% and APTT > 1.8 times control [2].

- **Surgery**

- In cases of hemorrhagic pathology, such as ruptured ectopic pregnancy, placenta previa, retroplacental hematoma and others, the surgeon will attempt to control the bleeding by compression or clamping, to allow restoration of effective blood volume and hemodynamics, before completing the rescue procedure. It may sometimes be necessary to change surgical techniques in order to rapidly address the origin of the bleeding: conversion to laparotomy during laparoscopic surgery, percutaneous surgery, endoscopic surgery, for example.

- In the case of non-haemorrhagic pathologies such as intestinal obstruction, peritonitis and the formation of the "third sector" and others, the intervention will consist of wide opening, treatment of the cause, peritoneal cleansing, drainage, aspiration and then closure in one or more planes.

- Surveillance

The standard monitocage alone provides a wealth of information, the relevance of which can be used to assess the situation:

- Blood pressure: taken every 5 minutes

Systolic blood pressure below 90, or even impenetrable, and sinus tachycardia (above 90 beats/min) indicate shock.

- Electrocardiogram: continuously monitored

Observation of the tracing enables us to monitor variations in heart rate, rhythm and conduction disorders, and cardiac distress with ST segment changes (sub-shift).

- Peripheral oxygen saturation curve: read continuously

It is a measure of tissue oxygenation, while desaturation may be synonymous with increased oxygen extraction due to acute anemia or hypovolemia.

- Temperature control: every 30 minutes

Hypothermia leads to hyper-viscosity of the blood, but also induces platelet adhesion disorders and bradycardia [17].

- Assessing the situation

We assess the situation by quantifying blood loss from the operating field, compresses and suction jar, and completing the biological work-up: CBC, platelet count, prothrombin rate, activated partial thromboplastin time, fibrinogen, blood ionogram, arterial blood gas, blood group and rhesus, hemoglobin and hematocrit levels. Samples should also be taken for blood culture if infections are suspected.

3-1-6 Evolution

The outcome is favorable if treatment rapidly restores blood volume and blood pressure. It is unfavorable if the initial treatment is ineffective, which may be due to the interplay of several mechanisms at the origin of the shock, to inadequate vascular filling or surgical hemostasis, or even to secondary complications due to organ failure, such as lesional pulmonary edema, acute renal failure, digestive hemorrhage, infections and others. In all cases, prevention of complications is essential.

3-1-7 Preventing complications

Severe shock is accompanied by ARDS and acute renal failure. Prevention of these complications depends on rapid correction of the shock.

Inhalation is possible in the event of severe upper GI bleeding in a shocked, obnubilated or exhausted patient. A gastric suction tube must be quickly inserted and the patient intubated to protect the upper airway.

Hemorrhagic shock leads to severe vasoconstriction in the splanchnic territory. This can lead to ischemic lesions of the digestive mucosa, which can be a source of bacterial translocation. Circulation in this area must be preserved by ensuring correct cardiac output, satisfactory perfusion pressure and improvement of local circulation through the use of dobutamine at 3 gamma/Kg/min.

3-1-8 Treatment of complications

In the event of renal complications, if anuria is less than 0.5ml-1ml/kg/h, fill the tank; if anuria persists despite filling, force diuresis with furosemide (lasilix*), the standard dose being 1 mg/kg/p [71].

In case of renal failure, go to 1 - 2mg/kg/h, then 1 to 2g per 24 hours at the ESF, until diuresis is restored. If this fails, dialysis is recommended.

If these measures fail, extrarenal purification should be considered.

3-2- ANESTHESIA IN OBSTETRICAL AND DIGESTIVE EMERGENCIES

3-2-1- Problems posed by the patient's condition

The history-taking process is designed to identify pathological conditions such as hypertension, asthma, diabetes, chronic bronchopneumonia, heart failure, etc., as unpreparedness increases the risk of decompensation of a pre-existing pathological condition.

A rapid somatic examination looks for edema of the lower limbs, jaundice and pale conjunctivae.

Whatever the clinical examination carried out, accurate assessment of renal and hepatic function, which requires a biological work-up, is not often possible in emergency situations in our hospitals.

- Assessing the current state

This involves assessing the disturbances caused by the impact of the hemorrhage or the third sector.

- Hemodynamic status

The situation most often encountered is cardiovascular collapse (systolic blood pressure below 80mm Hg) or shock (collapsed blood pressure with signs of visceral distress). Schematically, this may involve :

- a patient presenting with severe internal and/or external haemorrhage and severe anaemia. Signs include a thready pulse, collapsed blood pressure, profuse cold sweats, intense thirst, cold extremities and pale conjunctivae. The surgical condition in question may generally be polytrauma with significant hemorrhage, ruptured spleen, ruptured EPU, uterine rupture...
- of a patient presenting a picture of global dehydration with as signs': arterial hypotension, persistent skin fold, thirst, dryness of the underside of the tongue, hemoconcentration which is clinically translated by very colored palpebral conjunctivae, Foligo-anuria or amine ... the surgical condition involved may be peritonitis, intestinal obstruction ... [9, 53]

- Respiratory condition

Tachypnea is expressed either as hypoventilation or hyperventilation.

- Risks of pulmonary inhalation of gastric contents and a full stomach

Pulmonary inhalation of gastric contents (which are very often liquid) is responsible for pulmonary damage, the severity of which depends on the volume of liquid inhaled (volume greater than 25ml or 0.4ml per kilogram), the acidity of this liquid (PH less than 2.5) and its contamination by microbes. Oropharyngeal secretions and gastric fluid are reservoirs of germs. Contamination of inhaled fluid is a source of secondary superinfection, which can worsen the initial pulmonary damage. Pulmonary inhalation of acidic gastric contents leads to the classic MENDELSON syi-drome, a complication that can be avoided if the necessary measures are taken. Inhalation of gastric contents can be caused by a number of factors.

A full stomach is a situation where the classic preoperative lunch period has not been respected. The major risk of a full stomach is inhalation of gastric contents during induction of anesthesia or during recovery.

Factors that affect stomach evacuation are responsible for a full stomach. These factors are numerous:

- The type of food ingested: * High-fat foods prolong gastric emptying time: it often takes 8 to 10 hours for the stomach to be completely empty after eating these foods;

* High-sugar foods increase gastric acidity.

- Trauma, pain, anxiety, smoking and alcohol delay gastric evacuation. If the trauma or illness occurred a short time after the last meal, stomach evacuation may have ceased at that point. **It's safest to assume that any patient admitted in an emergency has a full stomach.**

- Medication: morphine drugs delay evacuation from the stomach and small intestine.

- Emergency digestive surgery (appendicitis, peritonitis, intestinal obstruction, etc.): these are sources of stomach fullness due to reflex or physical obstruction of digestive transit.

- Caesarean section, GEUR and obesity - Difficult intubation

Patients at risk of difficult intubation are at risk of inhalation due to the multiple aerodigestive tract stimulations that can occur during tracheal intubation attempts.

3-2-2- Induction agents [74]

3-2-2-1- Hypnotics :

Hypnotics with a short onset time of less than 45 seconds include thiopental, propofol, etomidate and ketamine.

Etomidate (0.3 mg/kg) and ketamine (2 mg/kg) have the advantage of preserving hemodynamic equilibrium in patients who are usually hypovolemic.

Propofol and thiopental: in the hypovolemic patient, they induce a reduction in blood pressure and cardiac output. If these agents are chosen for induction, their doses must be reduced (1.5 to 2 mg/kg for propofol and 3 to 4 mg/kg for thiopental) and the injection rate slowed.

In eclampsia, ketamine (which raises blood pressure) should be avoided and thiopental used [69].

3-2-2-2- **Curares**

Succinylcholine: this is the only curare with a short onset of action (of the order of one minute), proven efficacy in 99% of patients, and a short duration of action enabling rapid resumption of spontaneous ventilation in the event of intubation difficulties. In cases of eclampsia, it should be avoided, as it increases cardiac output abnormally during fasciculations, and vecuronium 0.1 mg/kg should be used to intubate the patient [69].

3-2-2-3- **Analgesics**

Fentanyl is still the most widely used drug in underdeveloped countries.

3-2-3- Anesthesia maintenance staff

There is nothing special or specific about emergency anesthesia maintenance. There are, however, certain aspects that need to be discussed.

Although nitrous oxide is formally contraindicated in cases of pneumothorax or emphysema, due to its diffusion in the closed cavities, this contraindication is only relative in cases of intestinal obstruction, since the digestive tract is further from the administration route and less well vascularized than the respiratory system. Only occlusions with significant gaseous distension should be avoided with nitrous oxide. Volatile agents (halothane, isoflurane, sevoflurane): all can be used to maintain anesthesia. In Caesarean section, halothane should not be used at a concentration higher than 0.5%, otherwise it may cause a reduction in uterine contractility, which is responsible for bleeding. What's more, high concentrations of halothane have a marked myocardial depressant and hypotensive effect, which can worsen the drop in blood pressure.

Curares (vecuronium, pancuronium, atracurium): these are all non-depolarizing curares. They are necessary for the management of abdominal emergencies, to achieve myorelaxation. The choice of curaie depends on the expected duration of surgery and associated pathologies (renal and/or hepatic insufficiency).

3-2-4- An example of anesthesia in shocked patients: emergency cesarean section for ruptured ectopic pregnancy

3-2-4-1- Conditioning the hemodynamically unstable patient

In an emergency, **pre-anaesthetic** care essentially consists of conditioning the patient, i.e. putting the patient in conditions that will enable him or her to undergo anaesthesia and surgery without major risk. Depending on the degree of urgency, care must be taken to correct any imbalance in a major vital function, such as respiratory function (for example, intubating the patient and giving oxygen) or circulatory function (perfusing in the event of arterial hypotension or dehydration), or preventing the inhalation of gastric fluid (nasogastric probing or administration of cimetidine 200mg orally).

In the event of an extreme emergency such as major haemorrhage (ruptured ectopic pregnancy, uterine rupture, stingray rupture, rupture of a large vessel, etc.), there's no time to lose. Immediate conditioning is essential, based essentially on :

- administration of oxygen at a rate of 4 to 6 *l* / min using a nasal cannula if the patient has difficulty breathing.

- fitting a good-calibre venous line, which must be firmly attached,

- request blood and rhesus grouping for a possible iso-group iso-rhesus blood transfusion, but while waiting for the transfusion, infuse ringer lactate or saline, or better still, a macromolecule (Haemaccel ...). In extreme emergencies, O-negative blood can be transfused to the patient, even if his or her blood group is not known. **This transfusion must always be preceded by a compatibility test which, when carried out correctly, consists of mixing a drop of donor blood with a large drop of patient blood serum, rather than a drop of donor blood mixed with a drop of patient blood** [52].

In other cases, such as severe global dehydration (peritonitis, intestinal obstruction), a distinction can be made between one to two hours, or even 4 hours, during which time the patient's condition can be ensured, based on :

- placement of a well-calibrated venous line, which must be securely attached, and infusion of lactated ringer lactate, 9% saline and 5% glucose serum. At least 2 liters can be filled before starting anesthesia. The sign on which to base the start of anesthesia in this case is a normalizing pulse. The main indication for vascular filling in emergency anesthesia is the correction of true hypovolemia due to hemorrhage, or relative hypovolemia due to reduced venous return to the heart as a result of vasoplegia;

- insertion of a urinary catheter to monitor diuresis in the event of overall dehydration. Normal adult diuresis is 1 ml/kg/hour. A patient suffering from peritonitis or intestinal obstruction should benefit from urinary catheterization and nasogastric catheterization, which will enable monitoring of the urinary and gastric fluid losses required for resuscitation.

- administration of cimetidine: 200 m g per os to reduce the volume of gastric fluid is necessary.

NB. In anesthesia, if a patient presents with a hemothorax, pneumothorax or pleurisy, pleural drainage must be performed prior to any anesthesia, even in an emergency [58].

3-2-4-2- Preparing anesthesia in the operating room

Before inducing anesthesia, it is essential to ensure that the anesthetic has been properly prepared. This preparation is based on :

- take a good-calibre venous line, which must be firmly attached, and start perfusion if this venous line is not taken during the preoperative resuscitation phase;

- preparation of intubation equipment, essentially including :

- laryngoscope in good condition, with batteries to ensure correct light ;
- a tracheal intubation tube of a size appropriate to the patient's size or age;
- a vacuum cleaner in good working order;
- and a suction probe.

Oxygen available in the operating room (wall-mounted oxygen, oxygen cylinder or oxygen extractor).

- preparation of products to be injected for general anaesthesia, such as :

- a benzodiazepine (diazepam);
- a hypnotic (thiopental) or (ketamine) ;
- a fast-acting curare (suxamethomam), for tracheal intubation;
- a curare for muscle relaxation (vecuronium);
- a centrally-acting analgesic (fentanyl).

All these products must be prepared in syringes. Each syringe must be labelled with the name and mass of the product per ml of solution.

Medications such as atropine (a parasympathytic), adrenaline and ephedrine (vasoconstrictors), should not be prepared in advance, but kept on hand for rapid use when needed.

▪ ensure that the respirator and multiparameter monitor are working properly, if available. **As part of anesthesia monitoring, the Pulse Oximeter is an indispensable instrument that must not be missed under any circumstances in the operating room.**

▪ check that you have a blood pressure monitor, a stethoscope, a small flashlight...

3-2-4-3- The per-anesthetic period

This period begins with the induction of anesthesia, passes through the anesthesia maintenance period and ends with the end of the surgical procedure. Pre-medication on the operating table, which is much more like pre-induction, takes place shortly before induction of anesthesia. In adults, this can be done with 5 to 10 mg diazepam IVD. Atropine is administered in doses of 0.5 to mg IVD.

- Induction of anesthesia

To begin induction of anesthesia, the patient must first be denitrogenated (or pre-oxygenated), i.e. oxygenated through a nasal cannula or face mask for at least 3 mm. This pre-oxygenation ensures that the patient has an oxygen reserve when anesthesia is induced. This is very important, because if a problem arises during induction of anesthesia, we have a few minutes to try and solve it.

During this pre-oxygenation phase, the patient's monitoring equipment is set up:

- the multiparameter monitor, if available;
- the blood pressure cuff on the upper limb, which does not have an infusion set;
- pulse oximeter on the thumb of the upper limb carrying the infusion set;
- and stethoscope.

Then we start by noting on the anesthesia sheet the various parameters that need to be monitored throughout the anesthesia:

- coloration of palpebral mucosa,
- SpO2,

- blood pressure,

- heart rate,

- respiratory frequency,

- diuresis and urine color,

- and temperature.

After denitrogenation for at least 3 min and when SpO_2 reaches 100%, several induction options may be available [69].

- In the case of general anesthesia (with ketamine) without intubation:

- induction is preceded by premedication on a pre-indrction table with ;

. IV injection of a benzodiazepine (dia/epam or mida/olam), which has the effect of attenuating ketamine-induced agitation, screaming or orrhea upon awakening ;

. and IV injection of atropine (parasympatholytic) to reduce ketamine-induced salivary secretions.

- the induction itself is carried out by injecting ketamine at a rate of 2mg/kg of the patient's body weight.

- oxygen is administered through a nasal cannula at a rate of 3 to 4 litres/mm.

NB. If ketamine anaesthesia is performed without intubation, a Guedel cannula should be avoided, as it may cause vomiting that can be inhaled.

- In the case of general anesthesia with intubation :

Induction may be preceded by tabletop premedication or preinduction (if the actual premedication has not been done before arrival in the operating room). We proceed with :

- IV injection of a benzodiazepine (diazepam or midazolam) which potentiates the effect of the hypnotic administered for induction;

- induction itself, which is achieved by IV injection of hypnotic (thiopental) or (ketamine);

- injection of a morphine (fentanyl) to prevent blood pressure from rising during intubation;

- injection of a slow-acting curare (suxamethonium, also known as celocurine) for tracheal intubation. Approximately one minute after curare injection, intubation is performed, and the tube is securely fastened after checking that it is correctly positioned in the trachea.

The elements of artificial or manual ventilation are put in place, with the administration of oxygen, anaesthetic gas (halothane) and nitrous oxide.

➢ **The maintenance phase**

This phase is marked by :

- Reinjection of products depending on the patient's clinical condition: injection of narcotic i/2 or[1] A of the induction dose if the patient wakes up,

. injection of analgesic if pain is present, usually manifested by a rise in blood pressure or agitation,

. injection of intermediate-acting curare (vecuronium) if muscle relaxation is required, as in abdominal surgery (only if the patient is intubated).

- Anesthetic gas can be inhaled at a concentration that depends on the patient's clonic state, and especially on his or her cardiovascular state if halothane is administered, which causes arterial hypotension.

- Vital parameters must be monitored every 10 minutes throughout the anaesthesia, and recorded on the anaesthesia record sheet, which perishes i to have the trend of the parameter curves showing the evolution of these parameters over time.

➢ **The awakening phase**

The awakening phase theoretically begins when the surgeon starts suturing the skin. The anesthetic gas (halothane) must be stopped, and if apnea persists due to a recent morphine injection, a morphine antidote (Narcan) must be injected. If apnea is due to a recent curare injection, the Prostigmine-Atropine combination must be injected.

The theoretical end of anesthesia coincides with the end of surgery. However, the anesthetist must monitor the patient until a satisfactory level of recovery is achieved. This should include effective spontaneous ventilation, allowing the patient to be extubated on the table before going to the recovery room.

3-2-4-4- The post-anaesthetic period

Theoretically, this period begins with the end of the surgical procedure. This is the period during which the products used to induce anesthesia are eliminated, allowing the patient to wake up or re-establish more or less normal breathing and circulation functions.

After the operating room, the patient is taken to the recovery room, also known as the post-interventional monitoring room (PIMR), where he or she is properly monitored to avoid complications such as dyspnea leading to apnea and then cardiac arrest, or a drop in blood pressure that could lead to severe shock.

Monitoring in the recovery room is based on discharge criteria from the post-interventional monitoring room (SSPI), which are based on parameters used to calculate the Aldrete score.

All incidents and accidents occurring during anesthesia are recorded in the anesthesia record, which is a medico-legal document.

3-3-CATEGORIZATION OF EMERGENCIES

Depending on their degree of severity and time to treatment, emergencies in hemodynamically unstable patients can be grouped into absolute (UA) and relative (UR) emergencies, by analogy with the categorization of casualties. This concept is derived from triage operations carried out in disaster situations.

The Noto-Larcan - Huguenard classification defines cauterization criteria as follows [65]:

- Absolute emergencies (UA)

They include all extreme emergencies (EU) and first emergencies (UA), whose management is characterized by two attitudes:

- immediate life-saving measures to ensure adequate ventilation and hemodynamics.

- priority discharge for further treatment.

Examples of absolute emergencies in our context include: ruptured extra uterine pregnancy (REUP), placenta previa, retro placental hematoma (RPH), hemoperitoneum and peritonitis.

For Noto and Larcan [65], extreme emergencies (EU) correspond to pathological situations that lead to acute cardio-circulatory and ventilatory distress and whose management is immediate, whereas first emergencies (Ul) are those that require prior care before evacuation, otherwise vital distress will appear, thus transforming them into extreme emergencies:

- need for supervision during transport ;

- need for intensive surgical treatment or resuscitation within 5 to 8 hours.

Absolute emergencies must be dealt with within no more than 06 hours.

- Relative emergencies (RU)

They group together all second (U2) and third (U3) emergencies. Here you need..:

- simple gestures to stabilize lesions;
- more or less delayed evacuation without special supervision;
- a deferred surgical procedure with no risk to vital prognosis.

However, it is important to bear in mind that the boundaries between these different categorizations are not formal, as a relative emergency can turn into an absolute emergency at any time. However, a general view of these categorizations enables us to act quickly and make swift decisions.

CHAPTER 4: CONCEPTUAL FRAMEWORK

Definition

The conceptual framework or conceptual model is a structured mental representation of a reality. It is a mental image, a way of representing reality [79]. In nursing, the conceptual model is the idea we have of our discipline, of our role as professionals; it is, in fact, our way of seeing, of conceiving the nature of the service we render to society [48]. There are several conceptual models in nursing, the main ones being :

- Florence NIGHTINGALE's conceptual framework;
- Virginia HENDÈRSON's conceptual framework;
- Dorothy OREM's conceptual framework;
- Calista ROY's conceptual framework;
- Dorothy JOHNSON's conceptual framework;
- Abraham MASLOW's conceptual framework.

In our work, we used Virginia Henderson's conceptual model.

As with any pathology, the role of the technician is crucial in the management of hypovolemia in emergency general anesthesia, in terms of reception, diagnosis, treatment, monitoring and prophylaxis.

According to Virginia Henderson, the human being is a biopsychosocial whole with 14 fundamental needs:

In the pre-, intra- and postoperative periods, the anesthesia technician must keep in mind the anatomical-physiological and biosycho-social particularities of patients.

When faced with a hypovolemic patient undergoing surgery, according to Virginia Henderson, we can remember a few essential basic needs that Ton must satisfy:

1) Need to eat and drink
2) Need to avoid danger
3) Dispose of normally by all routes of elimination
4) Maintain temperature under normal conditions
5) Communicating

According to Virginia Henderson, "the role of the Nurse is to assist the sick or healthy individual in maintaining or regaining his health by performing those duties which he would perform himself, if he had the strength, will or knowledge to perform them, so as to help him regain his independence as rapidly as possible".

The technician must identify the patient's needs in order to maintain or restore balance and hemodynamic stability during and after the operation. To meet all these needs, the technician must be able to provide efficient and effective care, helping the patient to regain his or her independence as quickly as possible.

4-1- UNMET NEEDS

4-1-1- Need to eat and drink

The hypovolaemic patient has many problems. In our review of the literature, we saw that hypovolaemia can be absolute or relative to the aetiology, which can be dehydration or haemorrhage. Hence the need to compensate for losses either by enteral or parenteral route.

This is where the concept of vascular filling comes in. The aim of vascular filling is to normalize blood volume. If the degree of dehydration is not high, peripheral venous lines can be used. If the degree of dehydration is high, the anesthesiologist should place the central venous line, and the anesthesia technician controls the filling by measuring the central venous pressure. In addition, the technician must prepare the elements for PVC measurement, which are: the three-way tap, a graduated ruler with water level, a mobile manometer, a stand, the filling solutes and the felt-tip pen.

4-1-2- Need to avoid danger

The hemodynamically unstable patient must be protected from the deleterious effects of anesthetic drugs and signs of intolerance to fillers. To avoid hypotension or shock, induction in such patients should only be carried out after the patient has been filled. Bright light and noise should be avoided. Similarly, pressure points must be protected to avoid pressure sores and thromboembolic risks. It is important to quantify and record blood loss, diuresis and vital parameters.

Mendelson's syndrome should be prevented by rapid-sequence induction with Sellick's maneuver, not forgetting placement of the nasogastric tube and deep anesthesia, always asking for the time of the last meal. And any failure or disturbance of vital parameters must be reported to the Anesthesiologist.

4-1-3- Need to eliminate normally by all routes of elimination

The elimination of waste products by the body is a sign that the body is functioning properly.

The anesthesia technician must check for anomalies through the urine bag, the diuresis, the bag receiving the liquid from the gastric contents. All these liquids must be noted on the patient's chart, which is a very important record.

4-1-4- Need to maintain temperature in normal conditions

Temperatures should be taken regularly to check for hypothermia and hyperthermia. The temperature should be recorded on the monitoring sheet.

4-1-4- Need to communicate with fellow human beings

Communication is important between the technician and the patient. It helps build confidence and inform the patient about all the procedures we perform, for example: finding the venous line, taking vital parameters, inserting the urinary catheter, denitrogenation and monitoring, so that the patient cooperates.

Our analysis model is as follows:

Table II Analysis model

Requirements	Events	Satisfaction	Intervention	Dimension	Component	Indicators
Eating and drink	- Drought in mucous membranes -Thirst Signs of handkerchief - Dyspnea Conjunctives lightly colored	No satisfied	- Infusion - Beverages simple - Water and juice fruit	Quantity to specify	Ringer lactate Salted serum Gelatin Blood	- Pulse filants, 80 pulse per minutes Voltage arterial < 80 mm Hg - FC accelerated
Avoid the danger	Affected by integrity physical or psychological or both	No satisfied	Filling vascular : Labeling drugs - Opening of the room (Check list) Preparation tray intubation Monitoring the score d'aldrete	- Curve status to be specified	- Curve versus time - Light, water - Magill forceps - Laryngoscope	- interpretation of the curve of PVC - interpretation from the anesthesia
Eliminate normally	- Oligo anuria	Not satisfied	- Filling Administration a diuretic	Quantity of urine released in 24 h.	Urine collector in good condition	Hourly diuresis
Maintained - the temperature in the normal-condition (36.5°. 37.5°)	Hyperthermia or hypothermia	Not satisfied	- Administration a antipyretics or turn on the air-conditioning or wrap hot	Visit air conditioning brings the room temperature within conditions to specify	Covers hot, the air conditioning, medicines, 'the thermometer medical	Control of the temperature

Communicate to its similar	-Shock - Communication ineffective at level intellectual, sensorimotor or emotional	No satisfied	Calm anxiety patient Kinesis therapy language	Check flow rate verbal.	- Medication - Films - Tape recorder	- Glasgow - Interrogation

Conceptual framework diagram

Anesthesia and intensive care technician

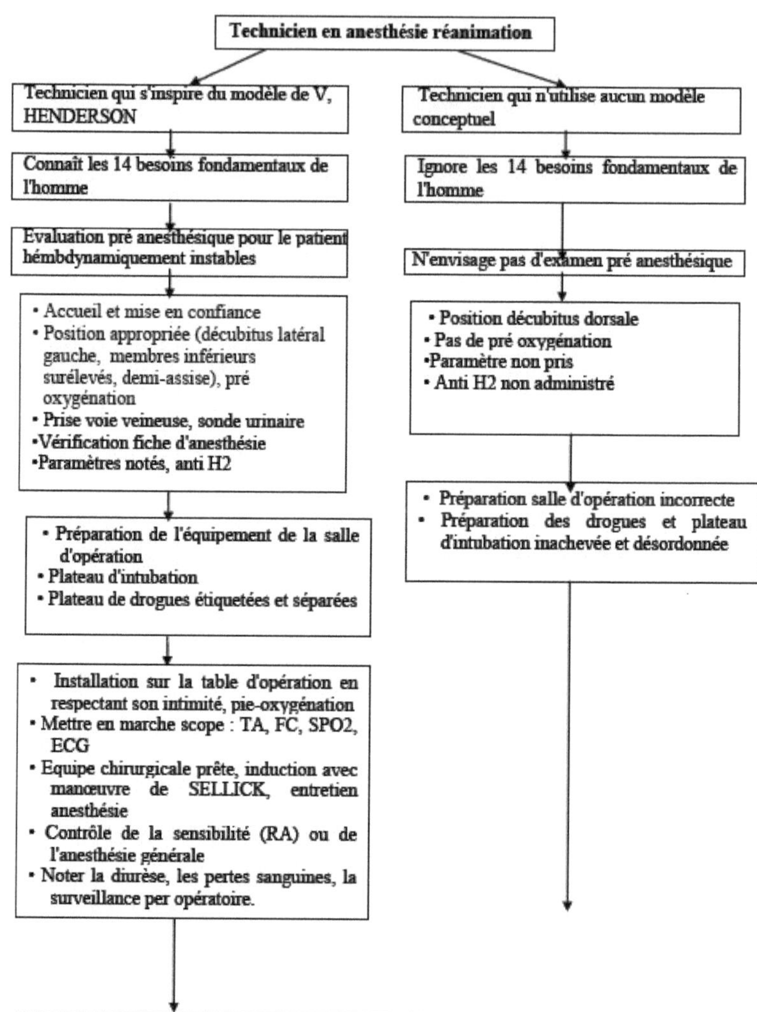

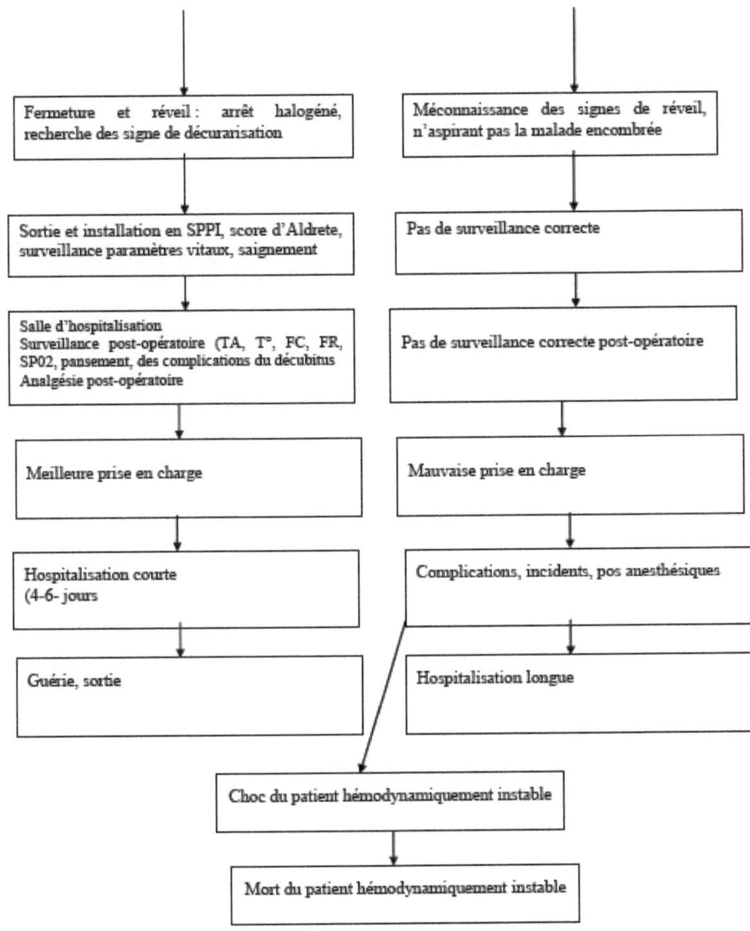

Figure 2 Conceptual framework diagram

4-2- OPERATIONAL DEFINITION OF CONCEPTS

- **Taking charge**: taking charge is an intervention designed to deal with a significant part or all of a person's problems [7].

- **Anesthesia** management: this is the process of dealing with a patient's problems in preparation for anesthesia. In practical terms, it involves consulting the patient in the pre-anaesthetic period, preparing the patient for anaesthesia, conducting the anaesthesia, and ensuring intra- and post-operative monitoring, avoiding and/or treating any complications [7, 11].

Incidents: these are small difficulties that arise during the course of a business [35],

Accidents: these are sudden, unforeseen events that cause damage, put people at risk, sometimes prolong hospital stays and increase costs [35].

Anesthesia: suppression of the sensitivity of an organ or of general sensitivity.

Hemodynamics: the study of blood movements and the forces that create them [26] or relate to the mechanical conditions of blood circulation (pressure, flow).

Hemodynamically unstable state: any patient with abnormal systolic blood pressure (SBP < 100 millimeters of mercury or SBP > 140 millimeters of mercury) and/or abnormal heart rate (HR < 60 beats per minute or HR 100 beats per minute).

Variation in PAS or HR: is equal to the difference between the highest intraoperative PAS or HR and the lowest intraoperative PAS or HR divided by the average of the two, multiplied by 100, hence the formula :

$$\Delta APAS = \frac{PASmax - PASmin}{\frac{PASmax + PASmin}{2}} \times 100$$

ΔAPAS = variation de pression, artérielle systolique
PASmax = pression artérielle systolique maximale
PASmin - pression artérielle systolique minimale

$$\Delta FC = \frac{FCmax - FCmin}{\frac{FCmax + FCmin}{2}} \times 100$$

ΔFC = variation de la fréquence cardiaque
FCmax= fréquence cardiaque maximale
FCmin = fréquence cardiaque minimale

Patients with potentially unstable hemodynamics: any patient with hemoperitoneum or a third sec our that could lead to hypovolemia as a result of hemorrhage or hydrolytic disorders.

CHAPTER 5: MATERIALS AND METHODS

5-1- TYPE OF STUDY

We carried out a retrospective, descriptive study on the files of patients operated on at the Yaoundé Gynaecological-Obstetric and Paediatric Hospital.

5-2- STUDY DURATION

Our work lasted 04 months i.e. from January 1er 2012 to April 30 2012. The study period was from l[ei] January 2011 to January 31, 2012 and concerned patient records.

5-3-STUDY LOCATION

This study was carried out at the Yaoundé Gynaeco-Obstetric and Paediatric Hospital.

This hospital, created in 2002, is the fruit of Sino-Cameroonese cooperation. It specializes in mother and child health care. HGOPY is located in the Ngousso district in the 5e arrondissement of Yaoundé, capital of the Mfoundi department and political capital of Cameroon. It is limited to :

- To the north, along the road linking the Ngousso district to the Etoudi and Manguier districts;
- To the south, speak of the Mfandena district;
- To the west, through the Etoudi district;
- A F East by Yaoundé General Hospital. This hospital offers the following services
- The administrative department (General Management, Secretariat, Accounting, General Supervision).
- Services include emergency, anesthesia-intensive care, gynecology, surgery and pediatrics;

FHGOPY's operating theatre consists of 6 operating theatres, including a maternity ward, and 5 large-surgery theatres. The latter are divided into a room for minor surgery, one for ophthalmic surgery and 3 others for other surgeries. Two post-interventional care rooms and the preoperative preparation room are annexed.

5-4-STUDY POPULATION

- **Inclusion criteria**

- Records of adult patients undergoing surgery.

- Records of adult patients operated on for obstetric emergencies (GEUR, hemorrhagic placenta previa, retroplacental hematoma, hemostasis hysterectomy, uterine rupture, postoperative hemoperitoneum).

- Records of adult patients operated on to form the 3ème sector (intestinal occlusions and peritonitis).

- Complete medical records.

- Non-inclusion criteria:

We have excluded :

- Records of patients operated on for corrective surgery.

- Records of patients under *15* years of age

- Missing or incomplete medical records.

5-5- SAMPLING

This was a non-probability consecutive sample, consisting of all patients operated on during the study period.

5-6- PROCEDURE

5-6-1- Pre-test

The pre-test was carried out in the intensive care unit of the Yaoundé Gynaeco-Obstetric and Paediatric Hospital.

5-6-2- Validity of the data collection instrument

It was validated by the dissertation supervisor, Head of the anesthesia and intensive care unit at the Gynaecological Obstetrics and Pediatrics Hospital in Yaoundé.

5-6-3- Building a research system

Based on operating theatre records, we identified cases of emergency laparotomy for pathologies likely to induce shock in the context of obstetric emergencies due to haemorrhage (ruptured ectopic pregnancy, haemorrhagic placenta previa, retroplacental haematoma, uterine rupture) or digestive emergencies due to the formation of a 3ème sector (peritonitis, intestinal obstruction). Then, from the registers of the hospitalization services, we established their circuit. From the archives of these different departments, we collected these patients' medical records. Finally, these records were selected for study according to our inclusion criteria. From these files, we used a pre-designed form to collect data concerning the pre-anaesthetic consultation, preparation for the operation, intraoperative management, post-operative prescription and patient outcome.

5-7- VARIABLES STUDIED

We studied the following variables.

- age,
- anesthetic risk through ASA classification
- anesthetic technique
- preoperative hemodynamic status through HR and BP
- the degree of urgency, through the categorization of emergencies (absolute urgency: extreme urgency and first urgency); relative urgency (second and third urgency).
- Quality of venous lines (type of venous line used, central or peripheral; number of venous lines inserted; size of catheters used)
- parameters monitored intraoperatively (ECG, PANI, SPao2, diuresis, temperature)...
- intraoperative blood loss (ECG, PANI, SPao2, diuresis, temperature)...
- intraoperative monitoring through
- anesthetic drugs used for anesthetic induction
- anesthetic drugs used for anesthetic maintenance
- the quality of filling solutions and blood products used
- duration of anesthesia (time between anesthetic induction and discharge from the operating room)
- duration of the procedure (time between incision and parietal closure)
- intraoperative incidents and accidents
- prescription of postoperative instructions f effective drafting of postoperative prescriptions, postoperative check-ups prescribed, prescription of prophylactic LMWH)
- patient outcome (stability or mortality).
- Intraoperative hemodynamic variations through intraoperative variations in systolic blood pressure (SBP) and heart rate (HR).

(The variation in PAS or HR is equal to the difference between the highest intraoperative PAS or HR and the lowest intraoperative PAS or HR divided by the average of the two, multiplied by 100).

$$\Delta APAS = \frac{PASmax - PASmin}{\frac{PASmax + PASmin}{2}} \times 100$$

ΔAPAS = variation de pression, artérielle systolique
PASmax = pression artérielle systolique maximale
PASmin - pression artérielle systolique minimale

$$\Delta FC = \frac{FCmax - FCmin}{\frac{FCmax + FCmin}{2}} \times 100$$

ΔFC = variation de la fréquence cardiaque
FCmax= fréquence cardiaque maximale
FCmin = fréquence cardiaque minimale

This variation was statistically significant if P (the plus value) was greater than 0.05. According to the ANOVA text, variance homogeneity occurs when P is greater than 0.05 [60,73], hence the formula :

$$P = \frac{m_1 - m_1}{\sqrt{\frac{\delta_2^1}{n_2} + \frac{\delta_2^1}{n_2}}}$$ For independent samples

m_1 = average of first sample

m_1 = average of second sample

δ_1 = standard deviation of first sample

δ_2 = standard deviation of the second sample

P = capital gain

Variations in systolic blood pressure > 25% of the initial value were considered significant. The same applies to heart rate.

5-8- MATERIALS USED

To carry out this retrospective work, we used a material comprising:

- computerized data collection sheets,
- service registers
- medical records
- Office equipment :
  - reams of paper, ballpoint pens, rulers, pencils, erasers, etc.),
  - computer equipment (computer, USB keys, CD Rom, printer).

5-9- STATISTICAL DATA PROCESSING

Results were analyzed using Epi Info version 6 and Microsoft Office software, in particular Excel 2007. Quantitative variables were studied by calculating averages and percentages, then presented in histograms and tables. Qualitative variables were described by calculating proportions and percentages, then presented in pie charts, tables, curves and histograms.

5-10- ETHICS

- The files used were exploited with the utmost discretion.
- The information collected is used exclusively for scientific purposes.
- The study required the approval of the national ethics committee: a letter was sent to the Chairman of the Cameroon Ethics Committee.
- An investigation authorization was sent to the General Manager of the Yaoundé Obstetrics and Pediatrics Hospital.

CHAPTER 6: RESULTS

➢ **Sample presentation**

From January 1[el] 2011 to January 31 2012, out of 606 patients undergoing emergency surgery, we recorded 231 shocked patients, operated on for obstetric and digestive emergency pathology, i.e. 38.11% of surgical emergencies, for which we made a breakdown of emergencies by month (Table III).

Table III Breakdown of emergencies by month.

Month	Number of surgical emergencies	Number of cases at risk of shock
January 2011	54	19
February 201 1	57	20
March 20 11	60	23
April 20 11	48	14
May 20 11	49	22
June 20 11	38	1 1
July 20 11	43	20
August 20 11	33	12
September 20 11	41	18
October 20 11	55	18
November 2011	37	19
December 20 11	51	17
January 20 12	40	18
Total	**606**	**231**

These 231 patients at risk of shock were operated on for gyneco-obstetric or acute abdominal hemorrhage.

In view of the large number of surgical emergencies, we divided patients according to surgical indications (Table IV).

Table IV Distribution of patients according to surgical indications

Surgical indications	Number of patients	Percentage (%)
GEUR	148	64,07
Hemorrhagic placenta previa	33	14,28
Peritonitis	18	7,79
Retroplacental hematoma	12	5,19
Hemostasis HRT	9	3,9
Uterine rupture	7	3.03
Intestinal obstruction	2	0,87
Postoperative hemoperitoneum	2	0.87
Total	**231**	**100**

Ruptured ectopic pregnancy was the main pathology likely to induce hemodynamic instability, with 148 cases (64.07%).

According to our inclusion criteria, we had a certain number of files selected for the study (Table V).

Table V Number of patients included in the study.

Surgical indications	Number of patients
GEUR	88
Hemorrhagic placenta previae	19
Peritonitis	16
Retro placent ire hematoma	05
Hemostasis HRT	05
Uterine rupture	7
Intestinal obstruction	2

Postoperative hemoperitoneum	2
Total	**144**

Of the 231 files meeting our inclusion criteria, we found 147, including 3 incomplete files which we excluded. In all, 144 files were retained for this study.

6-1- PRE-ANAESTHESIA CONSULTATION

6-1-1- Age distribution of patients

The mean age of patients was 29.68 years± 7.69 with extremes of 16 and 80 years (Figure 3).

Percentage of patients

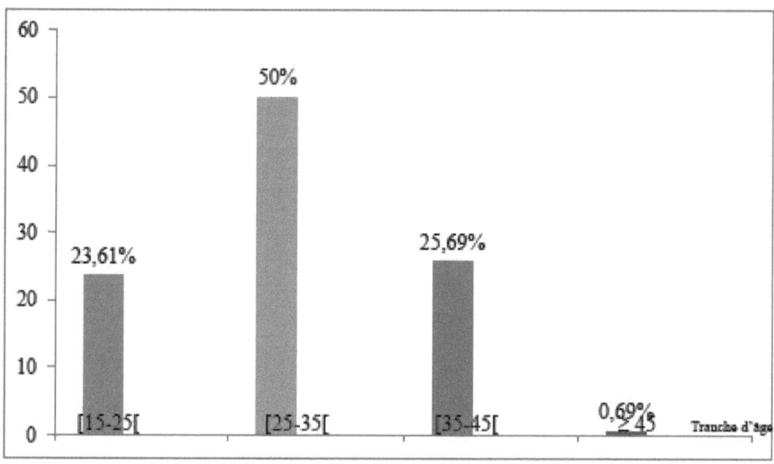

Figure 3 Distribution of patients by age

Half the patients (50%) were aged between 25 and 35.

6-1-2- Classification of patients according to ASAu

Figure 4 shows the American Society of Anesthesiologists classification.

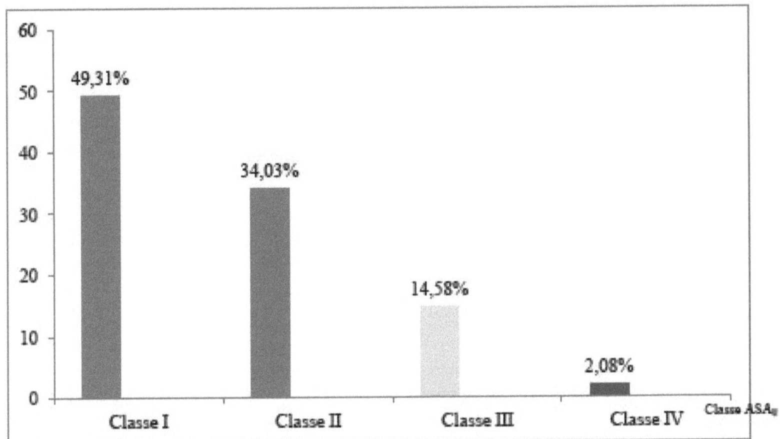

Figure 4 Distribution of patients according to ASA classification

ASA I patients accounted for the vast majority (49.31%), while ASA II patients represented 34.03%.

6-1-3- Altemeier patient classification

Patients were classified according to their septic risk (Table VI).

Table VI Altemeier patient classification.

Altemeier class	Number of patients	Percentage
Class I	/	/
Class II	95	65,97
Class III	31	21,53

Class IV	18	12,5
Total	**144**	**100,00**

In 65.97% of cases, patients were classified as Altemeier II.

6-1-4- Classification of patients according to degree of urgency

For the best management of hemodynamically unstable patients, we have categorized them according to degree of urgency (figure 5).

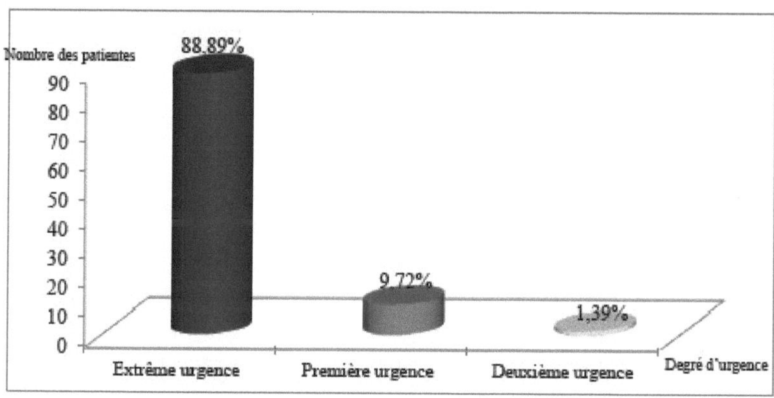

Figure 5 Classification of patients according to degree of urgency

88.89% of interventions were extreme emergencies.

Each consultation ended with an indication of the anesthetic technique to be adopted. We had 142 general anesthesias with orotracheal intubation and 2 spinal anesthesias (Caesarean section for hemorrhagic placenta previa and GEUR).

6-2- INTRAOPERATIVE CARE

6-2-1- Monitoring

The parameters monitored in all patients were: non-invasive blood pressure (NIBP); ECG; heart rate, Spo_2 and diuresis.

6-2-2- Venous approach.

In a harmonized manner, we determined the number of venous approaches placed in each patient (Table VII).

Table VII Number of venous approaches placed in each patient.

Number of venous approaches	Number of patients	Percentage (%)
1	1	0,69
2	138	95,83
3	5	3,47
>3	/	/
Total	**144**	**100,00**

In 95.83% of cases, two venous outlets were used.

6-2-3- Types of venous access used

From a technical and economic point of view, we assessed the type of venous approaches used (Table VIII).

Table VIII Types of venous approaches used

Type of venous approach	Number of approaches	Percentage (%)
Central venous catheter	/	
24 Gauge peripheral venous catheter (Cathelon G24)	/	/
Cathelon G22	08	2,74
Cathelon G20	32	10,96
Cathelon G18	245	83,90
Cathelon G16	07	2,40
Cathelon > G16	/	/
Total	**292**	**100**

Venous access was 83.90% with 18-gauge peripheral catheters.

6-2-4- Anaesthetic induction

Table IX summarizes the different hypnotics used for anesthetic induction.

Table IX Hypnotics used for anesthetic induction

Hypnotics	Number of patients	Percentage (%)
Thiopenthotal	63	44,37
Propofol	02	1,41
Ketamine	77	54,23
Etomidate	/	/
Total	**142**	**100,00**

Ketamine (54.23%) and thiopenthotal (44.37%) were the main hypnotics used for anesthetic induction.

- **Morphinics used for anesthetic induction**

Fentanyl was used for anesthetic induction in 137 patients (96.47%), and 5 patients (3.52%) received no morphine at anesthetic induction,

- **Curares used for anesthetic induction**

Table X Curares used for anesthetic induction

Curares	Number of patients	Percentage (%)
Vecuronium bromide	**51**	**35,92**
Succinylcholine then Vecuronium	**38**	**26,76**

Cisatracuriun	26	18,31
Succinylcholine then Cisatracuriun	11	7,75
Succinylcholine	16	11,27
Total	142	100,00

Vecuronium alone (35.92%) or preceded by succinylcholine (26.76%) was the main curare used for anesthetic induction.

- **Induction of spinal anesthesia**

The combination of Bupivacaine l0mg+Fentanyl 25µ ga was used in two young patients (25 and 30) with placenta previa and ruptured ectopic pregnancy respectively.

6-2-5- Maintenance of general anaesthesia

Anesthetics used for maintenance of anesthesia were represented mainly by Isoflurane and Halothane (Table XI).

Table XI Anesthetics used for anesthesia maintenance

Drug	Number of patients	Percentage (%)
Thiopenthotal	1	0,70
Ketamine	7	4,93
Isoflurane	96	67,61
Halothane	35	24,65
No	3	2,11
Total	142	100,00

6-2-6- Intraoperative monitoring

Patients' systolic blood pressure **at** induction averaged 117±25 mmHg. Heart rate at induction averaged 100±17 cycles per minute.

- **Hemodynamic status of patients at anesthetic induction**

The hemodynamic status of patients at anesthetic induction is shown in Table XII.

Table XII Hemodynamic status of patients at anesthetic induction

Hemodynamic instability	Number of patients	Percentage (%)
Hypotension (SBP<100mmHg)	17	11,81
Bradycardia (Fc<60/min)	/	/
Tachycardia (Fc>100mmHg)	49	34,03
Hypotension + Bradycardia	/	/
Hypotension+ tachycardia	11	7,64
Hypertension (PAS>140)	12	8,33
Hypertension + Bradycardia	/	/
Hypertension +Tachycardia	5	3,47
Total 1 (Hemodynamically unstable)	94	65,28
Normal PAS and normal Fc	50	34,72
Total	**144**	**100**

Ninety-four patients (65.28%) had an unstable hemodynamic state (abnormal systolic blood pressure and/or heart rate).

The mean change in blood pressure during the procedure was 34.39% ± 18.65, with a mean change in heart rate of 28.88% ± 17.95.

➢ **Variation in intraoperative PAS**

The change in systolic blood pressure (SBP) intraoperatively provided information on the patient's hemodynamic status (Figure 6). ≥ 30

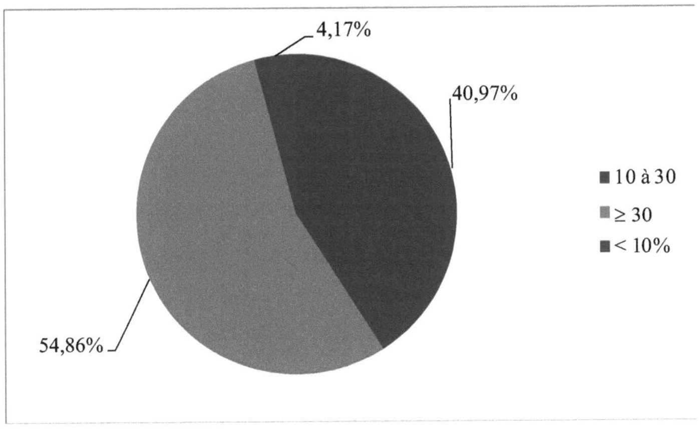

Figure 6 Variation in systolic blood pressure (SBP) intraoperatively.

The variation in intraoperative blood pressure was≥ 30% in 54.89% of patients.

- **Intraoperative variation in PAS according to the hypnotic used for anesthetic induction**

The intraoperative variation in PAS according to the hypnotic used for anesthetic induction enabled us to compare the relationship between Penthotal and Ketamine (Table XIII).

Table XIII Intraoperative variation in PAS according to **the hypnotic** used at induction.

Hypnotics	Variation	P
Penthotal (63 patients)	34,87±19,70	0,15
Ketamine (77 patients)	34,38 ±18,19	
Total mean change (144 patients)	34,39%±18,65	

The variation in PAS intraoperatively was not statistically different when penthotal or ketamine was used for anesthetic induction (34.87% VS 34.38%) P = 0.15 i.e. P > 0.05 according to the ANOVA test.

- **Intraoperative variation in PAS according to the hypnotic used for anesthetic induction**

Intraoperative variation in PAS according to the anesthetic used for anesthesia maintenance provided us with the best hemodynamic stability (Table XIV).

Table XIV Intraoperative variation in PAS according to the anesthetic used for anesthesia maintenance

Anaesthetic	PAS% variation	P
Ketamine (7 patients)	42,14±17,81	
Isoflurane (96 patients)	33,97±18,90	
Halothane (35 patients)	35,09±19,18	
Total mean change (144 patients)	34,39%± 18,65	0,94

Isoflurane produced the best hemodynamic stability, with a mean variation of 33.97%. There was a significant variation in PAS during anesthetic maintenance with ketamine (42.14%) $P = 0.94$ i.e. $P > 0.05$ according to the ANOVA test.

6-2-7- Intraoperative resuscitation

The fluids administered intraoperatively were crystalloids and colloids respectively (Figure 7).

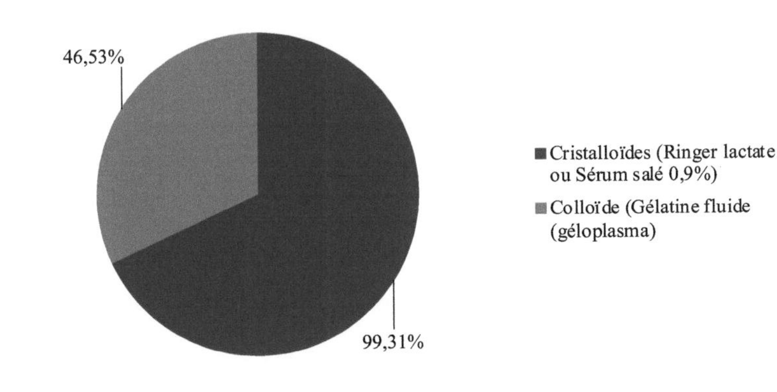

Figure 7 Quality of fluids administered intraoperatively

Intraoperative vascular filling with crystalloids was performed in 99.31% (143 patients) and 46.53% (67 patients) required colloids.

➢ **Quantity of fluids administered intraoperatively**

Patients received an average of 2425 ml ± 739 ml crystalloid intraoperatively and 337 ml ± 422ml gelatin fluid (Geloplasma).

➢ **Distribution of patients according to the quantity of crystalloids received intraoperatively**

We also divided patients according to the amount of crystalloid received intraoperatively (Table XV).

Table XV Distribution of patients according to the quantity of crystalloids received intraoperatively

Quantity (ml)	Number of patients	Percentage (%)
0	1	0,69
500- 1000	5	3,47
1500-2000	57	39,58
2500-3000	63	43,75

3500-40QO	17	11,81
>4000	1	0,69
Total	**144**	**100**

The majority (83.33%) of patients received between 1,500 and 3,000 ml of crystalloid intraoperatively.

- **Distribution of patients according to the quantity of colloids received intraoperatively**

The distribution of patients according to the quantity of colloids received intraoperatively enabled us to identify the different needs (Table XVI).

Table XVI Distribution of patients according to the quantity of colloids received intraoperatively

Quantity (ml)	Number of patients	%
0	77	53,47
500- 1000	63	43,75
1500-2000	4	2,78
>2000	/	/
Total	**144**	**100**

We note that 53.47% of patients did not receive colloids intraoperatively.

- **Transfusion of blood products**

Blood products were transfused in 40 patients (27.78%).

- **Quality of transfused blood products**

As there is no substitute for blood, the breakdown of blood products transfused was as follows (Table XVII).

Table XVII Quality of blood products transfused

Blood product	Number of patients	Percentage (%)
Red blood cells	24	60,00
Red blood cells and fresh whole blood	10	25,00
Fresh whole blood	6	15,00
Other	/	/
Total	**40**	**100,00**

The blood products transfused consisted mainly of packed red blood cells or fresh whole blood.

These patients received an average of 2 U of blood products, with extremes of one and five units.

- **Intraoperative blood loss**

Intraoperative blood loss was estimated at a mean of 1437 ml ± 877 ml.

6-2-6- Duration of surgery and anesthesia

Surgery time averaged 85.72 min ± 39.06 min, and anesthesia **time** averaged 101.13 min ± 41.76 min.

6-2-7- Intraoperative incidents and accidents

We noted one case of cardiac arrest during anesthetic induction of hemostasis hysterectomy for retroplacental hematoma in a 29-year-old patient with no previous history. This represents an incident prevalence of 0.69%. Lin external cardiac massage was performed, vascular filling with 2000ml Ringer lactate and 500ml gelatin fluid (geloplasma) with administration of adrenaline and atropine. The patient received 2 units of packed red blood cells and 3 units of fresh whole blood intraoperatively.

6-3- POSTOPERATIVE PRESCRIPTION

6-3-1- Intraoperative electrolyte fluids and transfusions

The average daily postoperative crystalloid prescription was 1732.64 ml ±585.11 ml.

Only one patient received colloids postoperatively (500ml gelatin-fluid).

Twenty-seven patients (18.75%) were transfused postoperatively, mainly with packed red blood cells.

6-3-2- Antibiotic prescription

Table XVIII Antibiotics prescribed

Antibiotics	Number of patients	Percentage
Clavulanic acid + amoxicillin	108	75%
Ceftriaxone + gentamicin + metronidazole	16	11,11%
Ampicillin + gentamicin + metronidazole	5-	3,4f%
Others (ciprofloxacin)	15	10,41%
Total	**144**	**100%**

This table shows that 75% (108) patients received the combination of clavulanic acid and amoxicillin as antibiotics.

6-3-3- Prescription of analgesics

Painting XIX Painkillers prescribed

Analgesics	Number of patients	Percentage
Paracetamol + tramadol + n.orphine	4	2,7%
Paracetamol + tramadol	26	18,05%
Tramadol + Diclofenac + Paracetamol	34	23,61%
Tramadol + Diclofenac	12	8,33%
Metamizol sodium + Morphine	1	0,69%
Diclofenac + Paracetamol	2	1,38%
Metamizol sodium+ tramadol+ Ketoprofen	31	21,52%

Metamizol sodium + tramadol	15	10,41%
Paracetamol + tramadol+ Ketoprofen + Morphine	9	6,25%
Novalgin+ Ketoprofen + acupan	1	0,69%
Metamizole sodium + Ketoprofen	2	1,38%
Tramadol alone	2	1,38%
Paracetamol alone	1	0,69%
Metamizol sodium + Paracetamol+ Tramadol+ Ketoprofen	4	2,77%
Total	**144**	**100%**

The most frequently prescribed analgesic was the triple combination (Tramadol + Diclofenac + Paracetamol) in 23.61% of patients.

6-3-4- Prevention of stress ulcers

Stress ulcer prevention was systematic in all patients and consisted of 73% ranitidine (azantac), 17% cimetidine and 10% omeprazole.

6-3-5- Prevention of thromboembolic disease

Thrombo-embolic disease was prevented in all patients by early lifting, wearing varicose stockings and prescribing Enoxaparin as early as 8ème hours post-op.

6-3-6- Post-operative monitoring of patients

- All patients were monitored in intensive care immediately postoperatively.

6-4- EVOLUTION

We noted no deaths in the operating room or in the post-interventional care room.

Table XX Distribution of patients according to length of hospital stay and disease progression

Length of hospital stay / Evolution	J0-J10	J10-J20	J20 and +	Total	%
Healing	80	40	22	142	98,61%

Deaths	1	0	1	2	1,38%'

Two cases of death (1.39%) occurred postoperatively in patients aged 34 and 36 respectively on postoperative days 8eme and 38^{ene} after laparotomy for peritonitis.

CHAPTER 7: DISCUSSIONS

7-1- STUDY LIMITS

Our study is limited by the problems posed by retrospective studies:

- incomplete and inadequate files,
- registers not containing all the data in the data sheet,
- archiving system that makes excavation difficult,
- these omissions introduce bias into the data collection.

7-2- PATHOLOGIES AND THEIR INCIDENCE

In our work, GEUR represents 64.07% of cases and is the main pathology likely to induce hemodynamic instability. NOTO. R [65] placed placenta previa at the top of the list. DADAO F [22] found a fairly stable incidence of retroplacental hematoma (5 per 1000 pregnancies in its severe form), while hemorrhagic placenta previa was estimated to occur in 1% of pregnancies.

7-3- AGE

The age group between 25 and 35 represents 50% in our study. This is the preferred period for good motherhood and intense sexuality, hence the plethora of ruptured ectopic pregnancies. However, well-monitored prenatal consultations help to avoid a variety of complications: GEUR, retroplacental hematoma, hemorrhagic placenta previa and others. This age range (25 - 35 years) was equivalent to the sample of Maurice LAMY 144 cases [46] and GOUIN 144 cases [35]. This age is also comparable to that of BALAGNY et al [5], who found an average age of 20 years corresponding to cases of post abortal sepsis.

7-4- ANESTHETIC CONCLUSION

- **Score Alteimeir :**

It can be used to assess septic risk.

In our study, 65.97% of patients were Alteimeir II. This is easy to understand, given the distribution of pathologies according to incidence.

Indeed, Alteimeir II patients benefit from a short course of antibiotics (48 hours maximum). However, in our sample of ruptured ectopic pregnancies, which very often have salpingitis caused by intracellular germs, some authors recommend putting these patients on antibiotics postoperatively. This adapted antibiotic therapy acts on intracellular germs (chlamydia).

- ASA classification

Several classifications have been proposed, the most important of which is the American Society of Anesthesiologist (ASA) classification.

The risk increases from class I to class V [67].

The majority of hemodynamically unstable patients were ASA 2 (49.31%) or ASA 1 (34.03%). These figures are similar to those of Léonard L. et al. who consider these to be subjects with a full stomach [52, 53].

- Degree of urgency

By analogy with LARCAN's classification [65], we have divided the pathologies encountered in our study into different degrees of urgency. This classification enabled us to assess the vital prognosis and understand the need for immediate treatment.

Encountered in 88.89% of cases, absolute emergencies were by far the most frequent, in line with the study by DESMONTS J-M, who states that 15.5% of anaesthesias in France are performed as emergencies, and the majority are performed on hypovolaemic or haemodynamically unstable patients [25]. This can be explained by the unpredictable nature of some of these conditions, such as ruptured extra uterine pregnancy, retro placental hematoma, placenta previa and peritonitis. In addition, ASA_U I patients who presented with an extreme emergency at the outset may be aggravated on the ward.

7-5- ANESTHETIC TECHNIQUE

In the emergency context, patients are generally on a full stomach, with a high risk of inhalation syndrome. This is why general anesthesia with orotracheal intubation is applied.

- The pre-operative fasting period is often observed.

- Pain, physical trauma and stress slow down digestive transit. The risk of inhalation is high. In our study, 98.48% of patients underwent general anesthesia with orotracheal intubation. This is in line with the CUMMINSRO étal. sample. [21].

However, 1.38% or 2 patients received spinal anaesthesia for Caesarean section with haemorrhagic placenta previa and GEUR respectively. In this context of obstetric and digestive emergencies in shocked patients, spinal anaesthesia is not indicated because of the vasoplegia it causes. However, it would be important to use pre-established protocols.

7-6- INTRAOPERATIVE MANAGEMENT

The intraoperative period consisted of :

- opening of the operating room;
- welcoming and settling the patient ;
- conditioning ;
- conducting induction ;
- maintenance of anesthesia and preoperative resuscitation ;
- recovery and transfer to the post-operative care room.

❖ **Opening of the operating room, reception and installation**

In France, it is governed by the Decree of 05 December 1994 and the Order of 03/10/1995 [66].

Preparing the anaesthetic site involves drawing up a checklist. In our study, it was difficult to verify the systematic use of the checklist, reception and installation, as this was a retrospective study.

❖ **Conditioning [52]**

It consisted of :

- two large-calibre peripheral venous lines for rapid and easy administration of solutions and anesthetic products. In our study, 95.83% of patients benefited from the placement of two venous ports.
- parameters monitored in patients included: blood pressure, respiratory rate, saturation, electrocardiogram, diuresis;
- antacid premedication with sodium citrate;
- keeping the vacuum cleaner within easy reach;
- the presence of helpers before the induction phase begins.

❖ **Conducting induction [54]**

It was marked by crush induction, which involved effective pre-oxygenation to ensure a sufficient supply of oxygen in the lungs to cover the period between anesthetic induction and placement of the intubation tube. This is followed by the **Sellick maneuver**, which involves exerting pressure on the cricoid cartilage prior to induction, in order to control regurgitation of gastric contents into the pharynx [54]. This is why the anesthesia technician must be cautious to avoid anesthesia-related incidents and accidents during induction, in line with the studies carried out by Tiogo C. et al. in Yaoundé in 1997.

7-7- DRUG ADMINISTRATION

This corresponds to the actual induction of general anesthesia.

However, intravenous hypnotics in anesthetic doses: ketamine at 54.23% and penthotal at 44.37% were the hypnotics used for anesthetic induction. However, etomidate hydrochloride is the most indicated molecule in states of hemodynamic instability, as it provides a good pharmacokinetic and pharmacodynamic balance. However, this molecule is not available in the underdeveloped world. However, ketamine is used in this indication because of the hemodynamic stability it provides, and because it is cheaper and more readily available. Thiopental is less hemodynamically unstable than propofol, especially when administered at low concentration and slow speed.

For intubation dose curares, vecuronium bromide at 35.92% or preceded by the administration of celocurine at 26.76% was the main curare used for anesthetic induction. However, in anaesthesia with a full stomach, a crush induction should be performed with a depolarizing curare such as suxarnethonium (celocurine*), with a short duration of action. Then, after intubation, administer a curare with a medium duration and delay of action, such as vecuronium bromide (norcuron*). However, celocurine is not widely available in our hospitals, whereas vecuronium bromide is currently less expensive and more widely used in our country.

After intubation, anesthesia was completed with the administration of morphine. A nasogastric tube was inserted if this had not been done preoperatively, followed by intra-anaesthetic resuscitation.

7-8- ANESTHESIA MAINTENANCE [75]

It is based on:

- narcosis was maintained with 67.61% isoflurane. In fact, isoflurane was the most available halogen and maintained good hemodynamic stability, unlike halothane, which more often than not ran out of supply.

- reinjection of curares as required for muscle relaxation during surgery,

- maintenance of analgesia through morphine re-injections,

- ventilation control,

- filling and loss compensation,

- monitoring of tracheal tube position, cuff pressure, saturation and gastric and oropharyngeal suctioning were required [75].

7-9- INTRAOPERATIVE MONITORING

- Systolic blood pressure

Indeed, blood pressure measurement is an essential part of anesthesia monitoring, whether general or locoregional. Interpretation of joint changes in blood pressure and heart rate can be used, among other things, to diagnose hemodynamic instability, over- or under-anesthesia [25, 28].

- Hemodynamic status of patients at anesthetic induction

The effects of anesthesia on blood pressure regulation: 25 years ago, Bristow showed that anesthesia depresses baroreflex control of heart rate in humans [53]. This study model has made it possible to evaluate the effects of virtually all anesthetic agents. In our study, 74 patients (65.28%) were hemodynamically unstable, and the variation during the procedure was 34.39% ± 18.65, with a mean heart rate variation of 28.88% ± 17.95.

Beyond that, the variation in intraoperative blood pressure was > 30% in 54.86% of patients. Similar results were obtained with intravenous anesthetics. Thiopental and propofol were less detrimental to baroreflex control of heart rate than were halogens. Ketamine and etomidate have very modest effects.

The baroreflex response changes throughout the operative period. In our study, the change in systolic blood pressure intraoperatively was not statistically different when penthotal or ketamine was used for anesthetic induction (34.87% vs. 34.38%).

- Intraoperative variation **in** systolic blood pressure depending on the anesthetic used Halogens have a concentration-dependent depressant effect. Halotane is the most depressant halogen, followed by enflurane and isoflurane.

In our study, isoflurane produced the best hemodynamic stability, with a mean variation of 33.97%, and there was a significant variation in PAS during ketamine maintenance anesthesia (42.14%).

The most obvious consequence of the depressant effects of anesthesia on blood pressure regulation is a reduction in bleeding tolerance. The depressant effect of anesthetics on the baroreflex should therefore be feared in terms of its functional integrity [25].

7-10- INTRAOPERATIVE RESUSCITATION

- Intraoperative fluid and electrolyte intake

Absolute hypovolemia is higher than relative hypovolemia, as observed by most authors. This is consistent with etiologies of hemorrhagic origin, dehydration or both, requiring fillers such as Ringer's iactate, blood, Geloplasma, saline and others [16, 45, 67].

When the aetiology is both haemorrhagic and due to dehydration, Ringer's Iactate and geloplasma are administered, depending on the degree of hypovolaemia, while waiting for blood to arrive [46]. Obtaining blood requires testing and appropriate monitoring. The quantity of crystalloids (Ringer Iactate) consumed was 2425 plus or minus 739ml intraoperatively and 337 plus or minus 422ml of gelatin fluid. The majority (83.33%) of patients received between 1,500 and 3,000ml of crystalloid intraoperatively. We note that 53.47% of patients did not receive colloids intraoperatively. Blood transfusion consisted mainly of packed red blood cells or fresh whole blood. These patients received an average of two units of blood products, with extremes of 1 and 5 units.

7-11- INCIDENTS AND ACCIDENTS

We noted one case of cardiac arrest during anaesthetic induction for haemostasis hysterectomy on retroplacental haematoma in a 29-year-old patient with no previous history, giving an incident prevalence of 0.69%. External cardiac massage was performed, vascular filling with 2000ml Ringer lactate and 500ml gelatin fluid (geloplasma) with administration of adrenaline and atropine. The patient received 2 units of packed red blood cells and 3 units of fresh whole blood intraoperatively [25].

7-12- AWAKENING AND EXTUBATION [6]

The risk of inhalation persisted after induction and was also present during the awakening phase. BARTHOLOMEUSZ et al have shown that, in both adults and children, inhalation occurs more frequently during extubation than during induction.

For this reason, extubation was performed under the following conditions:

- intraoperative emptying to reduce the volume of gastric co/itenu,
- complete awakening,
- state of total decurarization,
- antagonizing curarization at the slightest doubt when all these conditions were met. The patient could already be extubated by carefully aspirating into the mouth and, if possible, placing the patient in a lateral position.

7-13- POSTOPERATIVE PERIOD

The immediate postoperative period was marked by patient management in the post-interventional care room. Awakening is a critical phase, during which almost half of all anesthesia-related accidents occur [76], as TIOGO observed in 1997 [76].

Because of the risks associated with the residual effects of anesthesia, the consequences of the procedure performed, and pre-existing pathology that may arise during the first few hours following a therapeutic and/or diagnostic procedure under general anesthesia, continuous post-intervention monitoring is necessary [76].

In France, Decree 94-1050 of December 05, 1994 legally establishes the obligation for continuous monitoring after the intervention in a post-interventional monitoring room, as noted by KANS Field et al during incidents involving endotracheal intubation [42].

- A good installation

The lateral position facilitates the outward flow of secretions from a liquid in the oropharynx. The same applies to the dorsal decubitus position, with the head turned to one side.

Other parameters such as blood pressure, heart rate, diuresis, ECG, venous lines, drains, dressing, temperature, pain and abdominal circumference were regularly monitored.

Among the tests proposed to assess the degree of recovery of vital functions, the Aldrete score is the most widely used [15].

An Aldrete score of 10 is required to discharge the patient from the post-interventional care room and transfer him or her to the intensive care unit, gynecology department or surgery.

In all cases, post-operative care prescribed by the anesthesiologist was monitored.

7-14 POSTOPERATIVE PRESCRIPTION

- **Postoperative fluid intake and transfusion**

The average daily postoperative crystalloid prescription was 1732.64 ml ±585.11 ml.

Only one patient received colloids postoperatively (500ml gelatin fluid). Twenty-seven patients, i.e. 18.75%, were transfused postoperatively, mainly with packed red blood cells. This is a reminder of the frequent problems of anesthesia for hemodynamically unstable patients [10, 69].

- **Antibiotic prescription**

In our study, 75% (108) of patients were treated with amoxicillin + clavulanic acid [71].

- **Prescribing analgesics**

The most prescribed analgesic treatment was the triple combination (Tramadol + Diclofenac + Paracetamol) in 23.61% of patients. This is in line with the WHO's concern to establish a scale of analgesics [7].

- **Preventing stress ulcers**

Prevention of stress ulcers was systematic in all patients and consisted of 73% ranitidine (azantac), 17% cimetidine and 10% omeprazole. According to studies by J. ZE MINKANDE et al, the digestive manifestations of stress appear very rapidly following a variety of stressors, including severe illness, acute trauma and the postoperative period. This condition is seen in 2 to 10% of patients in intensive care [68].

- **Preventing thromboembolic disease**

Thrombo embo ic disease was prevented in all patients by getting up early, wearing varicose stockings and prescribing Enoxaparin from the 8^{erre} postoperative hour. Indeed, during the first Cameroon thrombosis control day on February 29, 2012 in HGOPY, J. ZE MINKANDE et al. again placed great emphasis on the prevention and treatment of venous iromboembolic disease in general surgery. Immobility, bed rest, paralysis of the limbs, etc. are all risk factors for venous thromboembolism in patients who are often neglected [1].

➢ **Patient monitoring**

All patients were monitored in the intensive care unit in the immediate postoperative period, and nursing care was provided (mouth care, perineum care, skin care, mobilization, nutrition, pressure sore prevention, etc.).

7-15- PATIENT OUTCOMES

As soon as we receive these patients, the procedures performed according to the pathologies in our context should follow, namely:

Surgical procedures in the operating theatre and medical procedures in the intensive care unit and maternity ward. The evolution of these pathologies was marked by 142 cures (98.61%) and 02 deaths (1.38%).

This means that the management of hemodynamically unstable patients at the Yaoundé Gyneco-Obstetric and Pediatric Hospital is prompt, appropriate and adapted to the emergency situation, thanks to the introduction of the minimum package, which is an emergency kit comprising the drugs and consumables needed for the immediate management of a patient in the operating room and intensive care unit.

However, it should be noted that the low death rate seems to be linked to a lack of archiving, with the loss of certain files or incomplete files not mentioning the course of the disease. This is one of the biases of retrospective studies.

CHAPTER 8: CONCLUSION AND RECOMMENDATIONS

8-1- CONCLUSION

This work has enabled us to gain a general overview of anesthesia in shocked patients in the context of obstetric and digestive emergencies **at the Gynaeco-Obstetric and Paediatric Hospital in Yaoundé.**

The essential pathologies that caught our attention were listed and categorized. For obstetric emergencies, they included ruptured ectopic pregnancies, hemorrhagic placenta previa and retroplacental hematomas, hemostasis hysterectomy, uterine rupture and hemoperitoneum. Digestive emergencies included intestinal occlusions and peritonitis.

GEUR was the main pathology likely to induce hemodynamic instability.

Half the patients were aged between 25 and 35.

The majority of patients were ASA I or II, and 88.89% of procedures were extreme emergencies.

The parameters monitored were: ECG, non-invasive blood pressure, heart rate, oxygen saturation, and diuresis.

GA was the main anesthetic technique and 65.28% of shocked patients were in the context of obstetric and digestive emergencies.

No deaths in the operating room

Management influenced by the absence of certain anaesthetic and blood products.

8-2- RECOMMENDATIONS

In view of the results of our survey and with a view to making our contribution to the management of shocked patients in the context of obstetric and digestive emergencies, we draw up the following proposals:

Ministry of Public Health:

- organize regular in-service training for staff
- provide each referral hospital with an emergency kit for the immediate care of shocked patients in obstetric and digestive emergencies.

- Supply hospitals with etomidate and blood banks with platelet concentrates and fresh frozen plasma.

To HGOPY General Management:

- organize anesthetic record keeping
- set up a computerized archiving system to provide a good database for future studies
- Maintain the monitoring equipment system

We are also encouraging a similar prospective study.

REFERENCES

WORKS

1. **Amina Wung, Jenerius A, Leke R.J. (2001).** *A case control study of ectopic pregnancies in Yaoundé,* Thèse de Médecine n°3741.

2. **Amstutz P, Guidet B, Simo-Moyo J, (1990).** *Perméabilité capillaire pulmonaire, le point sur la transfusion autclogue,* Arnete éd, Paris, 1 vol: 257- 270,

3. **Andem, (1997).** *Remplissage vasculaire au cours des hypovolémies relatives ou absolues,* SFAR; 5 (4), l^ère^ édition Paris, 3-6.

4. **Ayala et al, (1999).** *Hemorrhagic shock:* symptomatic treatment in a new perspective in intensive care.

5. **Balagny E. et al, (1993).** *Le remplissage vasculaire,* Arnette l^ere^ édition Paris, 30 - 35.

6. **Bartholomeusz Lucille, (2000).** *L'Anesthésie à moindre risque,* 2e edition, G mdin Road, printed in Côté d'Ivoire.

7. **Bekina K.F. (2008).** *Mémoire de fin d'étude. Evaluation de la prise en charge de la douleur au service d'accueil et des urgences de l'Hôpital Central de Yaoundé.*

8. **Ben Ammar M.S. et al, (April 2001).** *Journal Maghrébin d'Anesthésie-Réanimation et de médecine d'urgence N°31,* Volume 3, 79.

9. **Bengondo C, Ngoa S, Bengono G, (2001).** *Need of an oriented sensitization in teeth treatment at Yaoundé. Tropical Dent alJournal,* 38-40.

10. **Benhamou D, (1995).** Obstetrical anesthesia In: SAMUK : Anesthésie Réanimation Chirurgicale. 2^erne^ edition, Médecine-sciences, Flammarion, Paris; 719-739.

11. **Bernard and Geneviève P., (1989).** *Dictionnaire médical pour les régions tropicales,* République du Zaïre, Missionnaire de Saint Paul.

12. **Binam F, et al, (1997).** *Analyse situationnelle portant sur II03 anesthésies en zone défavorisée.* 9ème conférence médicale nationale, Yaoundé.

13. Brunner an suddarth's. (1999).Text copyright by, J-B - Lippincott company, New-York London Hagerstown, 979-980.

14. **Campbell MJ, Swinscow TDV (7009).** *Statistics and square one,* New York: Churchill Livingstone, 39.

15. **Carli P et al, (1991).***Urgences médico-chirugicales de l'adulte,* Maloine 2^cne^ édition Paris; 10-12.

16. **Carli-B. P. Riou, (1992).** *Urgences médico-chirurgicales de l'adulte,* Arnette edition, 2, rue Casimir Delavigne, 75006, Paris.

17. **Carpentier J. P., (2002).** *Soins Infirmiers aux urgences et en réanimation, transfusion sanguine n°21,* collections nouveaux cahiers de l'infirmière, 4e edition.

18. **Christophe Prudhomme, (2001).** *Déshydratation guide poche des urgences,* Maloine 2ème edition, Paris, 124-128.

19. **Clerel M., (1996).** *Air disasters.* In Catastrophes: de la stratégie d'intervention à la prise en charge médicale, **Huguenard P,** Edition Encyclopédie médico-chirurgicale, Poitiers, 541-553.

20. **Colliere M.F.,** *Soigner... Le premier art de la vie,* 2e édition Masson, Paris, Cedex, 2000.

21. **Cumminsro et al, (1991).** *Recommended guidelines for uniform reporting ofdataform out-of hospital cardiac arrest:* thé Utstein style circulation, 960-75.

22. **Dadao F, (2007).** *Epidemiohgie des urgences obstétricales à l'Hôpital Gynéco-Obstétrique et Pédiatrique de Yaoundé,* Mémoire pour l'obtention du diplôme universitaire de médecine d'urgence, 82.

23 **Davragon, (1984).** *Cahier de l'infirmière ; réanimation,* Ed. Masson.

24. **De Gaspen A, Narcisi S, Mazza E, Bettinelli L, Pavani M, Perrone L, Grugni CCorti A. (S.D).** 2 degrees Servizio Anestesia Rianimazione Trapianti Addominali, Ospedale NJguarda Ça Granda, Milano, Italy.

25. **Desmonts J-M., (1995).** *Risque anesthésique et accidents de l'anesthésie* in: SAMII K.: Anesthésie réanimation chirurgicale 2eme édition, médecine- sciences, Flammarion, Paris: 332-339.

26. **Ducassé J. Fuzier R, (1999).** *La prise en charge des malades dans les services d'urgence en 1998.* Actualité en réanimation et urgence, Paris, Elsvier, 255-269.

27. Duvaldestin PH. et al., (1989). *Second revised and expanded edition.*

28. **Egic, (1997).** *Grandes agressions et détresses médicales,* Masson 3e edition Pans, 51-63.

29. Engel BT and al, (2005). ***Laboratry*** *ofBehavioral sciences, National institute on aging, National Institutes of Health,* Baltimore, MD 21 224. CUIT opin crit care, 11 (3) : 264 -70.

30. **Fontanella J.M., Carli P. et al, (1993).** ***Les*** *matériels et les techniques de réanimation pré-hospitalière, les unités mobiles hospitalières des Samu,* édition Sgerm, collection médecine d'urgences Samu p. 126 - 127 - 167.

31. **Fortin M. F., (May 25, 1996).** *Processus de recherche:* de la conception à la réalisation, Décarie publisher, printed in Canada.

32. **François G., Carli P. et al, (1990).** *Réanimation et médecine d'urgence,* second edition, Masson, Paris.

33. **Gauthier P. Lafaye, (1990).** *Ane.thésie générale,* Masson edition, Paris, Milan, Barcelona, Mexico.

34. **Gines, P. Tito L, Arroyo V, Planas R, Panes J, Viver J, et al,** (1988). *Randomized comparative study of therapeutic paracentesis with and without intraveinous albumin in cirrhosis.* Gastroenterology, 94: 1493-504.

35. **Gouin F et al,** (1975). *Précis d'anesthésie,* 2ème édition Masson Paris, 286 -299.

36. **Grosclaude M.,** (2002). *Réanimation et coma, soins psychiques et vécu du patient,* Masson, Paris, Cedex 06.

'37. **Guidet B, Guerin B, Maury E, et al, (1990).** *Capillary leakage complicated by compartment syndrome necessitatind surgery.* Intern Care Mad, 332-333.

38. **Guyton GA, Lindesy WA, (1959).** *Effect of elevated left atrial pressure and decreased plasma protein concentration of tea development on pulmonary edema.* Cire Res. 619-657.

39. Harouna Y, Saidou B., (2000). *Les Perforations typhiques aspects cliniques thérapeutiques et pronostics.* Prospective study of 56 cases. Médecine d'Afrique noire: 47(6).

40 International Group for thé study of ascites in cirrhosis comparison of albumin, dextran-70 and hemaccel in thé prevention of effective hypovole°iia in cirrhotic patients with ascites treated with paracentesis. A randomized multiceriter study, part two (abstract). Hepatologyl995; 22:220A.

41. Kaboro **M. et al, (2005).** *Emergency anesthesia, Hôpital Général de Référence Nationale,* N'Djamena (Chad), 6.

42. Kans Field et al, (1990). *Incidence of blooding after oral endotracheal intubation. Anesthesiology,* 43-45.

43. **Kimessoukie E., (2008).** *A guide to learning the nursing approach.*

44. **King H. M. et al, (1988)** *Eléments d'anesthésie pratique,* Ârnette Paris, 30-40.

45. **Lamy M., (2005).** *Quand et quelle liquide prescrire en intraveineux,* 1ere édition Cedex Paris; 10-12.

46. **Lansac et al, (2002).** *Hypovolemia In: pratique de la P. V.C.* Collection pour le praticien, Masson Paris, 423 - 448.

47. **Laxenaire MC, Charpentier Cn Feldman L et al, (1991)** *Réaction anaphylactoïde aux substituts colloïdaux du plasma :* Incidence, facteur de risque, mécanismes, enquête prospective multicentrique française, ed, Fr, Anesth Réanim... 310.

48. **Legulluche T, Carsin H, et al (1989).** *Vascular filling in burn patients,* Réa, Soins intens, 331.

49. **Lemaire F., (1987).** *La ventilation artificielle n°4,* 2e tirage, collection d'anesthésiologie et réanimation.

50. **Lennon P, (1975).** *Conduite de l'anesthésie générale .Protocole du massachusetts général Hospital* Pradel 2ème édition, Pans, 209 - 219.

51. **Léonard L. Fareston et al, (2006).** *Clinical anesthesia manual, Massachusetts general hospital protocol,* 3eme Pradel edition.

52. **Lontchi Simo V.A., (2008).** *Final dissertation: anesthesiological management of the subject with a full stomach,* case of the Gynaecological Obstetric and Pediatric Hospital of Yaoundé, 60.

53. **Manelli J.C, Badetti C., et al, (1997).** *Réanimation et Anesthésie du brûlé,* Encyclopédie, Med, Chir, (Elsevier, Paris), Anesthésie -Réanimation.

54. **Maipeau, F. Sergent, B. Resil, E. Verspyck, B. Rachet, E. Clavier, (2004)** *Conférence d'actualisation, Congrès d'anesthésie et de réanimation,* Edition Elsevier, 624-634.

55. **MBU R, (2004).** *Topos de l'Hôpital Central*

56. **Moore F.D, (1966).** *Metabolic care of the surgical patient,* 1 vol, 1011P; W.B. Saundersco.) Philadelphia and London.

57. **Morin Y., (1997).** *Petit Larousse de la Médecine.* Edition Larousse Paris; 460.

58. **Moss GS, Cochin A, et al. (2011).** *Ejfects of saline and colloid solution on pulmonary function in hemorrhagic shock.* Surg Gyneco Obstet, 53-58.

59. **Ngah Ngah S., (2009).** *Bio statistique et épidémiologie,* Université Catholique d'Afrique Centrale, 3eme année licence.

60. **Nkoum B. A., (1999).** *Building, leading and managing a pedagogical project.*

61. **Nkoum B. A., (2009)** *De l'évaluation scolaire à l'évaluation des pratiques professionnelles en santé* ; thèse de Doctorat ; Université Aix-Marseille I - Université de Provence.

62. **Nkoum B. A.,** (2005). *Initiation à la recherche: une nécessité professionnelle,* Presses de FUCAC (PUCAC).

63. **Noto R, Huguenard P, Larcan A, (1994).** *Médecine de catastrophe,* Edition Masson, 228-241.

64. **Noumssi, (2010).** *Philosophie/Modèle/Démarche scientifique au cycle de licence en sciences infirmières,* 3eme année à l'Université Catholique d'Afrique Centrale à Yaoundé.

65. **WHO, (1998).** World Health Report 1998 Life in the 21ème century, a perspective for all, 167-168.

66. **Oxymag, (2005).** *Journal d'information professionnel des Infirmiers anesthésistes.* Edition Masson Paris; 25(85): 9-15.

67. Première journée camerounaise de médecine d'urgence et des catastrophes, 2005, du 24 au 25/11/2005 : 24.25.

68. SOU/DSMI-UNICEF project, **(January 2000**). *Obstetric anesthesia-intensive care protocol:* health center.

69. **Prudhomme C., (2003).** *Guide poche des urgences,* 2e édition Maloine, 3, 12, 46.

70. **Robert D., Robert M.et al, (1991).** *Oxygénothérapie de longue durée. Hypoxémie chronique grave,* published by Masson, Paris, Milan, Barcelona, Bonn.

71. **Saint-Maurice CL, (1992).** *Pharmacologie.* Volume II cours d'ISAR, Arnette edition n°5415, Printed in France.

72. **Sauvageon X, Viard P. (1994).** *Les produits de l'Anesthésie. Doin* Editeur 6, rue de Mézière 75006 Paris, 4-10.

73. **Schwartz D. (1996).** *Méthodes statistiques à l'usage des médecins et des biologistes,* 4^{en} edition, Flammarion.

74. **Simo Moyo J., Soh J., Afanc Ela A., (1996).** *Anesthesia and caesarean section: 50 cases at Yaoundé University Hospital,* Médecine d'Afrique noire, 411-416.

75. **Tiogo Christophe, (1997).** *Incidents et accidents liés à l'anesthésie à Yaoundé:* thèse médecine, Yaoundé.

76. **Tramer MR, (2001).** *A rational approach to the control of postoperative nausea and vomiting:* evidence from systematic review,

77. **Valleron A.J. (2007).** *Bio statistique,* Hammarion.

78. **Virginia Henderson. LE, M.A.** ***(1997).*** *Fundamentals of nursing,* Imprimerie Suisse. Geneva.

79. **Zarins CK, Rice CL, et al, (1982).** *Lymoh and pulmonary response to isobaric reduction in hemorrhagic shock.* AR Liss Inc, New York, 31-50.

REVIEWS AND ARTICLES

- **BELLOMO R, Uchimos.** ***Cardiovascular*** *monitoring tools:* use and misuse.

- **BIGATELLO LM Georges E. :** ***Hemodynamic*** *monitoring : Department ofAnesthesia and critical care,* Massachusetts general Hospital Harvard

- **JALONEN J.**: Invasive haemodynamic monitoring: concepts and practical approaches.': Department of Anaesthesiology, Turku university.

- **LOUGH ME.** *Introduction to Hemodynamic monitoring:* Diurnal variations in central venous pressure

- **MADGER** S, *How to use central venous pressure measurements:* M_c Gill, University Heald.

- Resolution n°005/2009 on the provisional management committee of the Yaoundé Gynaecological Obstetrics and Paediatrics Hospital.

- **WOODROW P.:** *Central venous catheters and central venous pressure.* Critical Care Intensive Therapy Unit, Kent & Canterbury Hospital, Easl Kent Hospitals NHS Trust.Philip.woodrow@kch-tr-sthames.nhs.uk.

- **GATES LM, Matthay MA:** *Central intravascular pressure measurements'.* Whent should we believe them?

- **WILSON M, Davis DP, Coimbra R.:** Diagnosis and monitoring of hemorrhagic shock during the initial resuscitation of multiple trauma patients: a review.

SITE

www.staartunisie.org/medias/pdf/mp_revue_31 .pdf. 2011/07/20

www.santedev.org/biblio/index-php.20/07/2011

www.refbooks.msf.org/MSF__Doco/Fr/clinical__guide/CG__fr.pdf. 07/20/2011

http://www.urgence-pratiquecom/2articles/medic/hemoiTage.htm. 15h45, 25/08/2011

http://www.infirniiers.com/etudiants-en-ifsi/coub/cours-reanimation-le-choc
hypervolemie.html.06/09/2011

APPENDICES

SHEET N°________________

PATIENT DATA

I- PRE-ANAESTHETIC CONSULTATION

1-1- Patient identification

Consultation date :

Preoperative diagnosis :

- Full name : ____________________________________ Age: ________________
- Gender: ________________ Occupation: _______________________________________

Marital Status: ____

-Intervention prévue :____

1-2- Antecedents

Medical: HTA Yes☐ No☐ Diabetes Yes☐ No ☐

Gastritis Yes☐ No ☐

Surgical Yes☐ No☐ Other specify __________________________

Gynaeco-obstetrics

G.P.____

Allergy Yes☐ No☐ Other specify __________________________

Toxicological Alcohol Yes☐ No☐ Tobacco Yes☐ No ☐

Autres préciser____

Transfusion Yes☐ No ☐

Anesthesiology Yes☐ No ☐

AG☐ RA☐

Autres préciser ____

Therapeutic Yes☐ No☐ Other specify__________________________

1-3- Physical examination

Vital parameters: weight (kg)_______ height (m)________ BMI______

Blood pressure:_____ Heart rate_____ Respiratory rate

General condition: conjunctivae: coloured□ pale□ very pale □

Dehydration: Yes□ No □

Asthenia: Yes□ No □

Weight loss: Yes□ No □

Intubation criteria

- Normal mouth opening (> 3cm) Yes□ No □
- Normal thyromental distance (> 6cm) Yes□ No □
- Mallampathi I□ II□ III□ IV □
- Dentition: Good□ Bad□ Dentures □
- Cervical mobility: normal Yes□ No □
- Prayer sign: Present: Yes□ No □

Cardiopulmonary examination

Normal systolic blood pressure (>100mmhg) Yes□ No □

Normal pulse (< 100 pul/min) Yes□ No □

Normal respiratory rate (< 20/min) Yes□ No □

SPO2 normal (> 95) Yes□ No □

Peripheral venous condition Good□ Mediocre□ Poor □

Varicose veins of the lower limbs Yes□ No □

Lower limb edema Yes□ No □

Normal cardiopulmonary auscultation Yes□ No □

Autres à préciser____

1-4- Preoperative paraclinical examination a) X-ray and electrophysiology

Chest X-ray: ____

-ECG:

____

_

-Ultrasound: -Scanner:

____

Autres à préciser____

b) Biological examination

Hemoglobin between (8 and 10) Moderate anemia Yes□ No □

(> 10) normal Yes□ No □

(< 8) Severe anemia Yes□ Name □

White blood cells: hyper leukocytosis Yes□ No □

Euleukocytosis Yes□ No□

Hypoleukocytosis Yes□ No □

Platelet: Thrombosis (<150,000) Yes□ No □

Severe thrombosis (<50,000) Yes□ No □

Moderate thrombosis (between 50,000 and 100,000) Yes□ No □

Mild tlirombosis (between 100,000 and 150,000) Yes□ No □

Prothrombin level (> 70%) normal Yes□ No □

Cephalin kaolin rate (< 40s vs. control) Yes□ No □

Normal urea Yes□ No□ High urea Yes□ No □

Normal creatinine Yes□ No□ High creatinine Yes□ No □

Blood glucose normal Yes□ No□ Blood glucose high Yes□ No □

Normal hematocrit Yes□ No□ High hematocrit Yes□ No □

Blood type and Rh requested Yes□ No □

1-5- Anesthetic conclusion

Alteimeir I□ II□ III□ IV □

Asa I□ II□ III□ IV □

Degree of urgency: scheduled□ emergency □

Autres à préciser____

Anaesthetic technique AG + IOT□ RA □

Autres à préciser____

II- PRE-OPERATIVE PREPARATION

- Fasting prescription Yes□ No □

- Resuscitation preparation Yes□ No □
- Antibiotic therapy Yes□ No □
- Ordering blood products Yes□ No □
- Quantity and quality to be specified in U/I____________________________________
  - Globular base Yes□ No □
  - Fresh frozen plasma Yes□ No □
  - Leaflet Yes□ No □
  - Red Globule Yes□ No □

III- PREMEDICATION

Ranitidine Yes□ No□ Quantity______________________________
Diazepam Yes□ No□ Quantity______________________________
Scopolamine Yes□ No□ Quantity______________________________
Autres à préciser____

IV- INTRAOPERATIVE CARE

Date de l'intervention____
_

Monitoring: TA______________FC ______________ EN ____________

ECG□ SPO $_2$□ Temperature □

PCV□ Others to be specified __________________________________

Venous lines and probes

Central line□ Peripheral venous line□ Number of lines_________

Gauge: G16□ G18□ G20□ G22□ G24 □

Urinary catheter□ Nasogastric catheter □

Intraoperative diagnosis: ____

Induction

Preoxygenation:□ _________________ SELLICK maneuver:□ _______________

Ketamine:□ _______________________ Celocurine:□ _______________________

Fentanyl:□ ____________________ B. Vecuronium:□

____

-Nesdonal : □ ____________________ Other drugs : □

____

Anesthetic care

* Reinjection of thiopenthal□ or ketamine □

* Isoflurane□ Halothane□ Fentanyl□ Other to be specified _____________

Mode of ventilation: Spontaneous□ Controlled: On ventilator□ Manual□

Intraoperative monitoring

- Highest intraoperative SBP ________________ mmhg
- Lowest intraoperative SBP _________________ mmhg
- Intraoperative hypotension (SBP <100mmhg) Yes□ No □
- Minimum heart rate __________min
- Maximum heart rate __________min
- Intraoperative tachycardia (>100PUL/min
- Intraoperative bradycardia (<60PUL/min□
- Minimum intraoperative saturation□ Maximum intraoperative saturation □

Intraoperative desaturation (<93%) Yes□ No □

Minimum intraoperative PVC□ Maximum intraoperative PVC□

Central venous hyperpressure (>5cmHO2) □

Central venous hypopressure (<OcmHO2) □

Minimum intraoperative temperature□ °C

Maximum intraoperative temperature. □ °C

Intraoperative hypothermia (<36°C)□ Intraoperative hyperthermia (>38°C) □

Diuresis at end of procedure: total quantity ______en ml

Flow ______en ml/kg/h

Intraoperative resuscitation

Intraoperative fluid and electrolyte intake

* Crystalloid: Ringer lactate or 9/1000 saline solution_________ml

* Colloid: Gelatin or geloplasma _________ml

* Antibiotic: Amorxicilin /Clavulanic□ _________ g

Ceftriaxone□ ________g

Gentamicin□ ________mg

Metronidazole□ ________mg

Cefuraxine□ ___________g

Ampicillin□ __________g

Others to be specified

____

Intraoperative transfusion Yes□ No □

Quantity and quality to be specified in U/I____

- Globular base Yes□ No □
- Fresh frozen plasma Yes□ No□
- Leaflet Yes□ No □
- Red Globule Yes□ No □

Preventive analgesia before incision

Ketamine before incision□ ____________________mg

Antalgic (preemptive analgesic): 1 hour to 30 minutes before the end of the operation

Paracetamol□ ________mg Novalgin□ _________mg Tramadol□ _________mg

Diclofenac□ __________ mg Acupan□ ______________mg

Wake-up and wake-up monitoring

- Table extubation Yes□ No □
- Intubated transfer to intensive care Yes□ No □
- Direct transfer to intensive care Yes□ No □
- Post-op care room monitoring Yes□ No □
- Trouvailles____
- Duration of anaesthesia ______________min
- Duration of surgery _______________min

V- POST-OPERATIVE PRESCRIPTION

1- Monitoring

BP□ Respiratory rate□ Heart rate□ Saturation □

ECG□ Consciousness□ Temperature□ Eva (pain)□ Abdominal circumference □ Diuresis □

Autres à préciser____

2- Medication

- Preventing stress ulcers:

  Ranitidine□ Cimetidine□ IPP □

- Antibiotic therapy or antibiotic prophylaxis:

  Amorxicilin /Clavulanic□ _______g

  Ceftriaxone□ _________g

  Gentamicin□ ________mg

  Metronidazole□ ________ml

  Cefuraxine□ ___________g

  Ampicillin□ __________g

  Autres à préciser____

- Analgesic

  Paracetamol□ _______mg Novalgin□ _________nig Tramadol□ ________mg

  Diclofenac□ _______mg Acupan□ _________mg Morphine□ __________ mg

Autres à préciser____

- Prevention of thromboembolic disease

Lovenox Yes☐ No☐ _____________mg

Autres à préciser____

- Hydration /24 hours

Crystalloids (RL or SS) _______________ml

Colloids (plasma gel) ________________ml

5% or 10% glucose serum with ________ml ions

5% or 10% glucose serum without ions ________ml

Autres à préciser____

- Prescription of compression stockings Yes☐ No ☐
- Prescription ck postoperative transfusion Yes☐ No ☐
- Para-clinical examinations prescribed postoperatively :

NFS ☐

Urea ☐

Creatinine ☐

Ionogram ☐

TP/TCK ☐

Others to be specified

____

- Postoperative nutrition :

Authorized☐ Yes☐ No ☐

Si Oui delay après intervention ________________________________en heure

VI- PATIENT OUTCOME OR COMPLICATIONS

____

____

NDE AZER Flavien
Etudiant Master II en Sciences de la Santé
Option Anesthésie -Réanimation au CSSS/UCAC
BP. 1110 Yaoundé-Cameroun
Tél. (+237) 22 22 50 56

Yaoundé, le 09/03/2012

À
MONSIEUR LE DIRECTEUR GÉNÉRAL DE L'HÔPITAL GYNÉCO-OBSTÉTRIQUE ET PÉDIATRIQUE DE YAOUNDÉ
S/C
CHEF DE SERVICE D'ANESTHÉSIE ET DE RÉANIMATION DE L'HÔPITAL GYNÉCO-OBSTÉTRIQUE ET PÉDIATRIQUE DE YAOUNDÉ

Objet : ***Demande d'une autorisation d'enquêter au sein de votre établissement hospitalier***

Monsieur,

Je viens très respectueusement auprès de votre haute bienveillance solliciter une autorisation d'enquêter auprès des malades de votre établissement sur le thème: **«ANESTHÉSIE POUR PATIENTS HÉMODYNAMIQUEMENT INSTABLES »**. Ce travail sera supervisé par le **Pr. ZE MINKANDE Jacqueline**, Chef de service d'anesthésie-réanimation.

Les informations recueillies nous permettront d'élaborer notre mémoire de fin d'études en vue de l'obtention du **Diplôme de Master en Sciences de la Santé**, option **Anesthésie-Réanimation.**

Dans l'attente d'une suite favorable, veuillez recevoir **Monsieur le Directeur Général**, l'expression de notre profond respect.

L'Étudiant

NDE AZER Flavien

Ci-jointe :

- La Clairance Ethique :
Autorisation n°084/CNE/SE/2012 du 02 Mai 2012

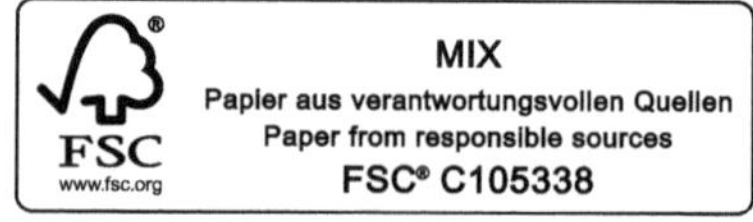

Printed by Books on Demand GmbH, Norderstedt / Germany